To Dwell in Your House

To Dwell in Your House

Vignettes and Spiritual Reflections
on Caregiving at Home

SUSAN FREEMAN

RESOURCE *Publications* • Eugene, Oregon

TO DWELL IN YOUR HOUSE
Vignettes and Spiritual Reflections on Caregiving at Home

Copyright © 2017 Susan Freeman. All rights reserved. Except for brief quotations in critical publications or reviews, no part of this book may be reproduced in any manner without prior written permission from the publisher. Write: Permissions, Wipf and Stock Publishers, 199 W. 8th Ave., Suite 3, Eugene, OR 97401.

Resource Publications
An Imprint of Wipf and Stock Publishers
199 W. 8th Ave., Suite 3
Eugene, OR 97401

www.wipfandstock.com

PAPERBACK ISBN: 978-1-5326-3243-3
HARDCOVER ISBN: 978-1-5326-3245-7
EBOOK ISBN: 978-1-5326-3244-0

Manufactured in the U.S.A.   10/12/17

For Phil Graubart, with love always

*Happy are those who dwell in Your house,
continually offering You praise.*

(Ps 84:5)

Contents

Acknowledgments | ix
Overview | xi

PART 1: VIGNETTES

I. Listening, Empathizing, and Being a Confidante | 3

II. Alongside Grief and Despair | 20

III. Attending to Fear | 33

IV. Overcoming Challenges to Connecting | 46

V. Navigating Changes, Boundaries, and Borderlines | 60

VI. Standing with Authenticity, Blessed with Revelation | 74

VII. Witnessing Growth and Discovery | 87

PART 2: REFLECTIONS AND THEORIES

VIII. Spiritual Pain: Theirs and Ours | 105

IX. To Be at Home | 109

X. What Can We Do to Serve? | 116

XI. The Most Potent Intervention | 120

XII. Anthroplogy of Listening | 123
XIII. A Theology of Listening | 128
XIV. Final Thoughts | 132

Bibliography | *133*

Acknowledgments

I AM GRATEFUL TO the patients and families I have had the privilege to serve as a professional chaplain; the inter-professional team members with whom I have collaborated, most recently at Sharp HealthCare; colleagues in the Association for Clinical Pastoral Education; the chaplain interns and residents I have taught over the last ten years; and members of my synagogue community, Congregation Beth El in La Jolla, California.

I am grateful, too, for the many individuals who encouraged me in this project—coworkers who listened to recordings of the vignettes and shared with me their responses and reflections; friends and colleagues who read a selection of the vignettes and provided helpful feedback and affirmation; and readers who sent me detailed notes with their suggestions.

I especially thank these individuals who read drafts of the manuscript and provided valuable input: Philip Graubart, Laura Michaels, Carol Freeman, and John Gillman. Mica Togami also provided consistent support throughout the project. Anne Wright edited each vignette prior to my sharing it with the staff and carefully edited the final manuscript. I deeply appreciate her generosity, professionalism, and friendship. I am grateful, too, to Ulrike Guthrie who provided professional editing and guidance along the way.

Acknowledgments

My family—husband, sons, sisters, nieces and nephews—is as loving and supportive as any person could hope for in a lifetime. I also lift up, with love and gratitude, the treasured memory of my parents, Joyce and Sam Freeman. I am extraordinarily blessed!

I thank Wipf and Stock for the privilege and honor of publishing my book with them.

Overview

INTRODUCTION TO HOME CARE VIGNETTES

In my role as chaplain and pastoral educator, I periodically share vignettes and reflections with my healthcare colleagues. My role on the caregiving team is to be especially attentive to and to address spiritual pain. Spiritual care visits I make to patients receiving home care services inspire the telling of these stories. Edited to protect my clients' identities, this book gathers together vignettes I shared with staff every couple of weeks over a period of approximately two years through a group voicemail that functions like a podcast. Because most of the clinicians spend their days out and about San Diego County visiting patients, we rarely see each other. By sharing these stories with my coworkers, I hoped to strengthen our connections with each other; offer support, encouragement, and reassurance; and ultimately to lift up the values and motivations that inspire us in our oftentimes demanding and solitary work.

In home care, I often engage with patients at critical crossroads in their lives—when they are trying to adjust to, make sense of, and cope with significant health challenges that affect their intimate relationships, finances, living circumstances, and spiritual worldviews. Many of the individuals I encounter may not be dying or ready to die, but the challenges in their lives make day-to-day

Overview

existence an entirely new, and sometimes daunting and incomprehensible, reality.

My home care colleagues are nurses, physical therapists, occupational therapists, speech therapists, health aides, social workers, and an extensive administrative support staff. I am in awe of the dedication, compassion, and care of this skilled group of individuals.

WE ARE ALL CAREGIVERS

All of us also have been recipients of care at some point in our lives—even if it was many years ago when we were children. For those of you reading who are professional caregivers, many of the circumstances described in the vignettes in this book will be familiar. What may be less familiar are reflections on how spiritual pain may affect those in our care.

While originally I wrote the vignettes for professional home healthcare workers, the topics and themes are relevant to anyone who has been in a caregiving role—whether as parents, siblings, sons, daughters, spouses, coworkers, or friends. Perhaps the most familiar caregiving roles are parents caring for young children, or adult children caring for aging parents Although spouses or life partners are typically first in line to care for each other when one or the other has an illness, there are plenty of other common configurations of caregiving. A patient I visited for two years had no living family, and a neighbor stepped up to be her main support. I've seen hired conservators become like family, fulfilling a caregiving role in the life of a physically or mentally vulnerable individual.

WHAT IS A SPIRITUAL CARE VISIT? WHAT IS SPIRITUAL PAIN?

A spiritual care or chaplain visit provides support to patients and/or their family members with respect for their beliefs, culture, and

OVERVIEW

values. Typically during a visit, a chaplain will help patients and their family members connect with their spiritual community, discuss their uncertainties and fears, and explore ways of coping with loneliness or disabilities. We also help them to discover what sustains them through illness and recuperation, express their feelings and thoughts, identify what gives them peace and meaning, pray or meditate with them, and/or reflect on their relationships.

HOW THIS BOOK IS ORGANIZED

Part 1 contains the vignettes, and part 2 presents theoretical and spiritual ideas.

Part 1: Vignettes

The book's first section presents thirty vignettes. Each one explores an encounter between me (the chaplain) and a patient(s) or patient's family member(s). I share various details and observations of the visits themselves, and then weave in reflections about these experiences. After each reflection, I offer a few tools for you to engage the vignettes at a deeper level:

- *Contemplations*—These are questions and suggestions for caregivers' own responses and reflections.
- *An Affirmation for Me*—This is a one- or two-sentence encapsulation of an essential idea presented in the vignette. Recalling the affirmation is a simplified way for caregivers to return to what may be meaningful inspirations or reminders.
- *A Prayer to Share*—These are words of consolation, comfort, peace, hope, love, faith, and encouragement that caregivers can choose to share with patients or their families. The prayer will reflect themes in the given vignette.

Overview

Part 2: Reflections and Theories

The second section of the book explores themes of spiritual pain, the meaning of "home," and different dimensions of listening. At the agency where I work, we include the offer of spiritual care to every patient as part of the intake process. Typically, however, home care agencies do not routinely offer spiritual care. My underlying objective in exploring the themes is to highlight the potential value of spiritual care to those receiving home care services. My reflections and teachings seek to illustrate how attending to spiritual concerns can be integral to the healing and well-being of those who are coping with a chronic illness, terminal health condition, or sudden health crisis. Part 2, also offers suggestions and concrete tools for providing compassionate emotional and spiritual support.

A NOTE ABOUT TRANSLATION

Introducing each "Prayer to Share" is a biblical verse. There is no single translation source represented in the pages that follow. Rather, I compared various sources, considered the original Hebrew, and constructed translations I consider best fitting for the context of this work.

PART 1

Vignettes

I.

Listening, Empathizing, and Being a Confidante

SPIRITUAL CARE TYPICALLY BEGINS with listening, empathizing, and being a confidante. Indeed, any good relationship requires these foundational elements. In the five vignettes that follow, the themes of intent listening, empathizing, and being a trusted confidante are front and center. Being an effective caregiver requires us to cultivate all these skills, and to return to them again and again to support and sustain the healing we hope to provide.

NELLIE: ENCOUNTERED ANEW

Those of us who provide care for others in their homes bring an array of skills, tools, and remedies to our encounters. A primary, easily overlooked gift we bring when visiting a person for the first time is the grace of seeing someone anew.

"Come on in!" the patient called out when I knocked on the door for my first visit. As I entered, a voice at the other edge of the room asserted, "I'm Naughty Nellie."

"Oh! That's quite a name!" I exclaimed. I was caught off guard by this woman's surprising and forthright way of introducing oneself. Naughty Nellie? Hmm. However, her tone was light and sufficiently humorous that I filed away the comment. We could come back to it later.

Eighty-three-year-old Nellie grew up Protestant, converted to Catholicism when she married, became detached from religion after she divorced, but retained her belief in God. The most pressing reason she was receiving home care was that nurses came several times a week to change bandages around her swollen legs. She also was on oxygen 24/7, had diabetes and numerous other health concerns. A more recent development was a breast cancer diagnosis. When I first visited, she had just started five weeks of five-days-a-week of radiation. This treatment would be followed by an MRI and likely surgery, and there were no guarantees that this intensive treatment would eradicate the cancer.

Her health situation sounded devastating to me, so I didn't expect the stream of affirmations she expressed with regard to all the good things in her life: the home care nurses who came and changed her bandages were wonderful; everyone was so good to her when she was at the hospital; the garden at the rehab place had a beautiful magnolia; the Meals-on-Wheels people made sure she had little, delicious fruit cups with each meal since her diabetes prevented her from having other sweets; the driver who took her to radiation treatments walked her *all* the way in to the building; the library had a generous program for lending her books, sending them by mail *at no cost*; she had a sweet, new great grandchild; and on and on. She also told me a long story about her disapproval of an old friend who did not seem to be fighting her cancer as aggressively as possible.

I wondered how I could be most helpful to her. It seemed this patient was finding coping strategies that were working for her. Even when I invited her to explore her feelings of loneliness, she quickly asserted that making phone calls and writing letters satisfactorily addressed this. I did notice a rushed immediacy in her responses to my questions and a defensiveness in her tone-of-voice, leading me to ask myself if her positivity was something new, something she was trying out on me. It was almost as if she didn't want me to "catch her" in negativity. When it came time to wind down the visit, I asked, "Is there anything else we should talk about?"

She said, "I'll tell you how I got the name Naughty Nellie." She went on to tell me that when she was a little girl, each week her mother gave her a penny in an envelope to bring to Sunday school for charity. Instead, she would tear open the envelope and buy candy. Thus, she received her nickname.

This *confession* of sorts—some seventy-five years later—may have been the essential impetus for her desire to see the chaplain. Having gotten this off her chest, we closed the visit with my offer to bless her. "Oh, I sure could use that!" she exclaimed. Perhaps a blessing today could begin to replace the curse that had attached itself to her since childhood. Nellie, at eighty-three years old, wanted to be seen anew, to be considered someone who could see the good, who could express gratitude, who had a strong will to live. She wanted me to see her for who she felt herself to be at her very essence. In listening to and blessing her, I could help her release that age-old label, the defeating self-image. Nellie was not naughty, but noble. With all the tools and skills we bring to our patient visits, there may not be anything as powerful and potentially healing—even redemptive—as seeing the good in the other, as allowing the other to be encountered anew.

Contemplations

- What experience have I had in my life in which I felt people did not see me for who I really am?
- What feelings did that elicit, and how did I process them?
- When have I discovered a "good" in another person that I had previously overlooked? What did I learn as a result?

Part 1: Vignettes

An Affirmation for Me

I can be someone who sees the good, who appreciates the good, and who commits to seeking the good.

A Prayer to Share

God saw all that God had made, and it was very good. Gen 1:31

I will turn their mourning into gladness; and give them comfort and joy instead of sorrow. Jer 31:13

> God, though the course of my life
> Can present hoops and hurdles,
> Struggles and convolutions,
> Underneath it all
> You assure me of my worthiness.
> You recognize the whole of me,
> My accomplishments, and my failures,
> My triumphs, and my disappointments.
>
> Thank You for granting me life,
> Seeing me wholly,
> Revealing to me such a full range
> Of Your expansiveness.
> Though in my life I have navigated
> Shadows and darkness,
> In Your compassion,
> You guide me to gladness,
> And show me the path to comfort and joy.
> Your goodness inspires me to
> Emulate and celebrate the good,
> The very good,
> With which You created me.

You ignite Your divine spark within me—
Light and bright,
I am a mirror of Your luminosity.

MADELINE: ARCHAEOLOGISTS OF FEELING

There are encounters that require extra patience and persistence for discovering what may be buried most deeply in the minds and hearts of those for whom we care. After two last-minute cancellations on her part, Madeline and I finally met on our third try. We sat down together in her small but tidy apartment. Madeline had been overwhelmed by all the changes in her life. Besides the challenges with her physical health, her home did not exactly feel like home. She had been living in the senior residence for just six months, having lived fifteen miles north, in her own trailer park home for the past twenty years. Three months into her stay at her new residence, eighty-seven-year-old Madeline had hip-replacement surgery. A few weeks into her recovery, she had a heart attack, returned to the hospital, and left with a new stent in place.

Madeline struggled with loneliness. In light of her health crises, she was unable to participate in the activities provided at the senior residence. Before her health issues, she had been an active member of her church, serving in a leadership role. Her church was now fifteen miles away and getting to any other church would be difficult because she was now unable to drive. Madeline also told me about Harry, her "significant other," as she called him, who also was on the other side of town. In talking about her loneliness and isolation, we discussed what resources might there be for her to reconnect with a spiritual community. We discussed each of her three daughters and their offers for her to move in with them. To do so, though, would require Madeline to leave San Diego, which she was reluctant to do. As we explored the pros and cons of moving in with one of her daughters, Madeline finally revealed the most profound source of her reluctance—leaving ninety-one-year-old Harry.

Part 1: Vignettes

Harry had been down to her new place just twice in six months because he didn't drive either. He had planned to move into the same residential complex as Madeline. But on the day that the papers needed to be signed, Harry demurred. Instead, he bought Madeline's former trailer home and stayed in the trailer park fifteen miles north. It was clear to me that Madeline remaining in the county for Harry was probably not going to provide either of them with the kind of emotional and relational support each needed, nor would just inhabiting the same county address any emerging needs for day-to-day physical care support. It had become dauntingly difficult for Madeline and Harry to see each other, let alone take care of each other's physical needs. Our visit gave Madeline a forum for expressing the pain that came with her realization that Harry was slowly disappearing from her life.

In working with patients at home, we see a great deal of loss. While certain losses—like deaths and divorces—are readily apparent, I find that at times we need to be like archaeologists. We need to strive to discover what is buried more deeply. When we invest in loving patience with those we tend, they may allow us to glimpse the heart of their grief, like a shard of a vessel that tells a much bigger story. We are archaeologists of feeling. When we take the time to understand the buried griefs, the hidden sources of pain, we are better able to help our patients to see a reconstructed vessel, to reimagine a vision of greater wholeness for themselves.

Contemplations

- When I feel lonely, how does that color the way I see the world?
- What helps alleviate loneliness?
- When have I assisted someone in easing the most severe edges of his/her loneliness?

An Affirmation for Me

When I take the time to understand the buried griefs, the hidden sources of others' pain, I become an archaeologist of feeling and can help others to see a reconstructed vessel, to reimagine a vision of greater wholeness for themselves.

A Prayer to Share

But the pot he was shaping from the clay was marred in his hands; so the potter formed it into another pot, shaping it as seemed best to him. Then the word of God came to me, saying, "Can I not do with you, Israel, as this potter does?" declares God." Like clay in the hand of the potter, so are you in my hand, Israel." Jer 18:4–6

>God, I am lonely.
>I have known many griefs;
>Some are present with me daily.
>I try not to grip them so tightly,
>But when, in my aloneness my life feels smaller,
>My griefs feel bigger.
>My life experiences shape me;
>But You shape me too.
>Remind me to let go of trying too hard,
>Remind me that I can become malleable—
>In Your hands.
>
>In Your hands,
>Help me to feel Your touch.
>You draw me out and contain me,
>An ever-changing vessel.
>As long as I remember
>That I expand and contract in Your hands,
>That you hold me precious,
>I can trust that You support and sustain me—

Part 1: Vignettes

To do what I need to do,
To be and become who I am meant to be.
I am ever changing,
And ever secure
In Your hands.

GENEVIEVE: MIRRORING EMPATHY

For Genevieve the emotional, spiritual, and physical challenges she faced ran painfully deep. During the initial year in which this forty-year-old mother of a three-year old was diagnosed and treated for cancer, her husband became ill and died.

In my third visit to Genevieve, she learned that the only recourse left to fight the new cancer metastasis in her body would be chemotherapy. This would be her third intensive course. Although she had many worries about enduring this demanding treatment once again, she lingered in confiding about the trauma of losing her hair. She remembered details from the last round, including how handfuls of hair would fall out while she showered, and the feelings she had about being bald and unattractive. As Genevieve's tears flowed, I was intently present to the many details of her experience, feeling great compassion.

In a quiet moment, hours after the visit, Genevieve's words replayed themselves in my mind. I didn't immediately notice that as I thought about her I absentmindedly was twirling the ends of my hair in my fingers. I only became aware of this subconscious action because of the soft strands of hair releasing themselves into my hands. In touching my hair a few more times, I discovered an atypical number of loose strands forming small clumps in my hands. I was astonished by this very concrete manifestation of my being touched by Genevieve's story. Although my experience was nowhere near the hair loss Genevieve was anticipating, my body was telling me that I empathized with her in ways I hadn't realized.

In recent years, there has been growing interest in the interface between spirituality and neurology. You may have heard of mirror neurons. Mirror neurons in our brains are shown to "light up" parallel to certain actual experiences of others. This mirroring can include empathy—on a certain level we can and do *feel* what others feel. What do we do with this? We healthcare workers know to be cautious about becoming overly invested or overly emotionally involved or enmeshed with our patients. And yet, science points to evidence that we humans are programmed neurologically to empathize—literally "to feel with."

I can think of a few strategies for how to embrace our capacity to empathize, while taking care that our empathy remains healthy and appropriate for our own well-being. The first is self-awareness—a willingness and an intentionality to see ourselves and the situation we are in honestly. A second is self-compassion—being gentle with ourselves when we find we are deeply touched by our patient encounters. A third is self-care—cultivating strategies for processing and releasing the suffering we encounter—whether it's debriefing with a colleague or counselor, writing in a journal, praying or meditating, engaging in physical activity, or something else.

One of my clinical pastoral education students shared with me a daily ritual she created for herself for when she returns home from the hospital. She has a glass jar filled with water. From a supply of pebbles, she chooses one to represent her experiences for the day. After reflecting on the experiences and honoring the feelings that arise, she drops the pebble into the water and lets go of the day's intensities.

Contemplations

- What are my own experiences with mirroring those I care for?
- How do I monitor self-awareness?
- How do I cultivate self-compassion?
- How do I practice self-care?

Part 1: Vignettes

An Affirmation for Me

When my felt sense of empathy "lights up" congruent with the actual experiences of those I serve, I am reminded of how profoundly connected I am with all human beings.

A Prayer to Share

Be holy, because I, the Eternal your God, am holy. Lev 19:2

Deep calls to deep at the sound of your waterfalls; all your waves and breakers have swept over me. Ps 42:7

> God, I am created in Your image.
> You call to me, and I respond.
> God of Strength,
> I am strong.
> God of Courage,
> I am brave.
> God of Hope,
> I trust.
> God of Peace,
> I am calm.
> God of Brokenness,
> I am broken.
> God of Healing,
> I heal.
> God of Forgiveness,
> I forgive and am forgiven.
> God of Love,
> I am loving and lovable.
> Your depth calls to my depth.
> You call to me, and I respond.
> You are, and thus I am.

LANCE: ACCOMPLICES TO PRAYER

When I met fifty-year-old Lance, I knew his situation was very worrisome. As he did not fully reveal just how close to the financial edge he was living, however, I didn't understand then the true precariousness of his circumstances. His health insurance was going to run out at the end of the month, he had missed several mortgage payments, there were no disability funds coming in, his wife was in jail, and he wouldn't be able to work for at least several months due to injuries following a rock-climbing accident. Although at the time I didn't have all the details of his finances, I understood he would benefit from the wisdom and resources of the social worker.

With that referral in place, Lance and I focused on other issues. We talked through the experience of the rock-climbing accident that had left his foot mangled and the surgeries and infections that followed. Lance's concern about his wife was foremost on his mind. Fretting about her was emotionally consuming. His loneliness grew steadily, in sync with the many hours he spent home alone. He had to rely on friends and neighbors to get to appointments because his foot injury prevented him from driving himself. Spiritually Lance was looking to God for comfort and guidance. He regretted not being able to get to church.

After meeting with Lance, social worker Kathy assessed that it would be nearly impossible for him to earn any income in the immediate future. She set out to investigate any creative way to find him enough funds to see him through the immediate crisis. With the unique complications of Lance's situation, the resources Kathy typically turned to would be limited. She had a thought. How about contacting Lance's church? Perhaps the congregation would have emergency funds for someone in a crisis situation. Kathy and I consulted about this and decided it was worth a try. After numerous exchanges with church leaders, Kathy indeed was able to secure a $500 check for Lance. In relaying the story to me and to the other clinicians working with Lance, Kathy was moved to tears by the generosity and compassion of Lance's spiritual community.

Part 1: Vignettes

In my post-$500-check visit with Lance, our conversation came round to discussing things he had learned as a result of his accident and its aftermath. He became emotional as he said that he learned that God answers prayers. He viewed the money he received from the church as God's vehicle for responding to his woes. Later, I thought a lot about this part of my interchange with him. Whether or not God answers our prayers is an age-old question. From the biblical Job to Mother Teresa, individuals have wrestled with what to believe about God's active engagement in our lives. Even if we assume the $500 check *was* divine intervention, on a practical level the money had to come from an earthly source—in this case from church members and a home care social worker motivated and committed to alleviating suffering.

When we are part of a community attentive to suffering or when we persevere in helping a patient or loved one avert a crisis, we become accomplices to prayer. Those who believe that God answers prayer still may wonder how, why, or when exactly this happens. From Lance's story, my discovery became that, no matter how one understands the workings of the cosmic realm, each of us can play a part in becoming an answer to prayer.

Contemplations

- What do I believe about answers to prayer?
- When was a time I felt I played a part in answering prayer?
- To what degree are "answers to prayer" dependent on human efforts?

An Affirmation for Me

When I am discouraged, I trust that answers are out there for me, not necessarily what I expected, but shedding light and providing guidance, nonetheless.

Listening, Empathizing, and Being a Confidante

A Prayer to Share

You answer us with awesome and righteous deeds, O God our deliverer, in whom all far off ends of earth and sea put their trust.
Ps 65:6

> God, over the years, I have called to You,
> Recently, maybe more than ever.
> My life seems to go off track, then on track,
> Off track again, then back to a semblance of equanimity.
> As my days and seasons cycle through hope and despair,
> And as I turn toward You and away, toward You and away,
> Your responses can feel elusive—
> Distant, then encouraging,
> Silent, then affirming.
>
> As I call to You now,
> Please help me to listen hard for Your answers:
> Open my ears to hear Your compassion,
> Open my eyes to see Your amazing creation,
> Open my heart to feel Your tender concern.
>
> As sure as birds twitter,
> Lizards scramble,
> Children giggle,
> A neighbor shows up, or
> Sweet, crisp apples ripen to perfection,
> I have learned, as You have taught me—
> Answers—awesome and righteous—
> Come from unexpected places.
> If I close my eyes in fatigue,
> If comprehending feels impossible,
> If my heart becomes weary,
> Still, you will answer:
> "Come, rest in Me . . . Come rest in Me."

Part 1: Vignettes

JAMES: CONFESSION

Following my visit to James, a forty-eight-year-old man recovering from hip surgery, I reflected on the process and power of confession. In our introductory phone call, James shared that he was in acute emotional pain. There were things he had done in his life about which he was ashamed. Being forced to slow down due to his recovery process had allowed thoughts and feelings of regret to catch up with him, triggering a downward spiral into despair and self-loathing.

Most religions have purification rituals in which a person may become spiritually cleansed, renewed, or metaphorically reborn. Concrete symbols, such as water, may help convey a sense of transformation, as in Christianity's use of water for Baptism. Other religions also use water for ritual immersions. Members of certain spiritual traditions ritually wash deceased members of their community, purifying the body as it departs this life, preparing it for the transition to whatever comes next.

A ritual purification process can be more abstract, too, with words rather than water as the tool for transformation. Formal processes for spiritual cleansing include a Roman Catholic priest hearing confession and granting absolution to his parishioner, or a Jewish worshiper emerging from reciting Day of Atonement prayers feeling renewed and restored. Alcoholics Anonymous lists confession as the fifth of its twelve steps to recovery, asking followers to admit "to God, to ourselves, and to another human being the exact nature of our wrongs." Coming clean at the end of life is an important final rite for many religious individuals.

When I arrived at James' home, we sat down, and he told me his story. While he did not affiliate with a specific religion, confessing his wrongdoings and his sorrowful regrets had become essential to him for progressing with his healing. Without cleaning out the wounds of his mind and heart, he was too depleted in spirit to direct effort toward healing his body. To repair his will to live and to thrive healthfully once again meant he had to first repair his soul.

At the conclusion of our visit, James shared how much better he felt. I imagine many of us hear similar responses from those who confide in us. They may tell us how helpful it is to be able to share their story, assuming we respond by carefully listening, respectfully helping them process feelings of regret, and supporting them in making the amends they have identified as being most healing for themselves and for those whom they may have hurt. Their words and body language may reflect how expressing the truth about who they are and what they have done—how "coming clean"—is integral to their willingness to embrace life and pursue health again.

Still, I wonder what exactly happens that can make confession a transformational experience. In other vignettes in this book, I address loneliness—how a deep and existential ache can plague those who spend hours on end by themselves and how this can have a deleterious effect on the body and spirit. Holding shame and regrets inside can be a kind of loneliness too. There's social loneliness and psychic loneliness. Psychic loneliness is when people feel alienated from others due to self-imprisoning sorrowful thoughts and feelings.

When we hear a confession, we affirm the opportunity for others to renew themselves, to return to purification and truth. In stepping into connection with those who are suffering with regrets and shame, we hold out the hope for healing from the debilitating strain of psychic loneliness. We lift up the possibility for transformation.

Contemplations

- When has a confession been healing for me?
- How do I feel when someone chooses to confide in me?
- How ideally might I respond to confessions of regrets and shame (assuming they do not involve unreported crimes)?

Part 1: Vignettes

An Affirmation for Me

Establishing relationships where others feel free to confess their deepest anguish allows me to offer consolation that healing of mind and spirit is possible.

A Prayer to Share

Then I acknowledged my sin to You; I did not cover up my guilt; I resolved, "I will confess my transgressions to God, and You forgave the guilt of my sin." Ps 32:5

> God, there is a lot I have done right in my life,
> But I also have regrets—
> Some come back to haunt me from time to time,
> To the point of my feeling enormously burdened.
> What could I have done differently?
> Why didn't I do things differently?
> How might I have hurt others?
> How have I hurt myself?
> I confess these burdens to You,
> Trusting that You know what to do with them.
> When hearts are open and vulnerable,
> Even broken,
> You hear confessions and forgive.
> I understand I must make amends where I can,
> That there is no statute of limitations on reaching out
> To those I may have hurt.
> But there also is no limit to my reaching out to You,
> And to Your reaching out to me.
> You see me for all I am.
> You see my wholeness—my flaws and my attributes.
> In creating me,
> You have given me the hope and reassurance

Listening, Empathizing, and Being a Confidante

That You will forgive,
that I am worthy of forgiveness,
that Your mercy is boundless.

II.

Alongside Grief and Despair

A CAREGIVING ROLE OFTEN includes journeying alongside individuals experiencing grief and despair. Some individuals may have experienced the recent death of a loved one. So many of those needing caregiving are in the later stages of life. While struggling with their own health issues, they may see the deaths of their spouse, life partner, or closest friends. When individuals get into their nineties, it is not uncommon for them to witness the deaths of their children, now in their seventies. As caregivers, we may find ourselves in the role of comforting and supporting those for whom we care through the process of mourning.

Of course, the experience of grief and despair is not limited to facing the deaths of loved ones. In caregiving, we likely will come across grief and despair around losses of independence, community involvement, mental acuteness, financial stability, changed (and strained) intimate relationships, and so on. Our challenge is to recognize grief and despair when we see them, be open to exploring patients' experiences around these difficult emotions, and walk alongside them as they process their feelings and discern how to move on with their lives.

MITCH: WAITING, HOPING

Although I'm not fluent in Spanish, I studied the language for enough years to be familiar with basic vocabulary. I've always been struck and a little puzzled by the verb "*esperar,*" meaning both "to wait" and "to hope." In spending time visiting Mitch, I became even more puzzled about it. For nine months, the sixty-nine-year-old Mitch had suffered from unrelenting leg pain that emerged following a botched surgery. In visit after visit, the home care team would hear him describe one "waiting" event after another: the wait to get a new pain prescription; the wait to see whether the new medication would work; the wait to receive a steroid shot; the wait to see whether another steroid shot would be allowable; the wait to see the surgeon again; the wait to see whether his insurance would allow a second opinion with a new surgeon; the wait to see a specialist at the pain clinic; and on and on.

How can a word (*esperar*) encompass the two experiences of waiting and hoping? For Mitch, each seemingly interminable stretch of waiting drained his hope—as if the two notions had nothing to do with each other!

In visiting with Mitch, what I discovered is that hope isn't one monolithic destination. Mitch and his home care team wanted to see him reach the destination of pain *relief*. In the meantime, how could the team members help him negotiate the emotional drain and discouragement in waiting?

One strategy was to support Mitch in exploring and embracing the "little hopes" that could sustain him through the waiting. "Little hopes" that Mitch and I explored were prayer, meditation, deep-breathing techniques, gratitude practices, strategies for improving his relationships with his daughters, and making the commitment to strengthen parts of his body that were not in pain. Of course there also was the hope that emerged when a member of the home care team would sit and listen open-heartedly and compassionately. With our visits, the patient began to dare to hope, to rally in enduring the wait. *Our* patience conveyed that the patient's experience was worthy of attentiveness and loving care.

Upon further reflection I recalled that the concluding lines from Psalm 27 also end with a word translated sometimes as "wait," and other times as "hope." The words are "wait for the Lord" or "hope in the Lord." The psalm then continues with the assertion that to wait/hope by looking to God is a means of cultivating strength and courage. To be less explicitly theological, we could say that exploring sources of growth and meaning beyond the confines of our most immediate pain can be a vehicle for living a more courageous life.

With regard to our role as caregivers, when we consistently show up for those for whom we care, wait with them, week in and week out, we convey the hope that whatever better future may be possible, we will pursue it. This powerful message weaves those two translations of *esperar* together and can provide much-needed courage to those we serve. It *is* possible to imbue waiting with hope.

Contemplations

- What strategies have I used to get me through the stresses of waiting?
- What "little hopes" have helped sustain some of the individuals for whom I've cared?
- What "little hopes" sustain me when I'm down?

An Affirmation for Me

In showing up week in and week out for those for whom we care, we convey the hope that we will pursue whatever better future may be possible.

A Prayer to Share

Wait for God; be strong and take heart and wait for God. Ps 27:14

> God, I'm waiting and hoping;
> Hoping and waiting.
> For better news, more options, new remedies;
> For freedom from medical appointments, side effects,
> Special diets, and tedious therapies.
>
> How my life will unfold in days to come
> Is a Mystery.
>
> Therefore, God of hope,
> With Your steadfast grace and graciousness,
> Remind me—
> To pour out my longings to You.
> I'm waiting for You,
> But You, also, are waiting for me.

DOLORES: FLAVORS OF TEARS

Dolores is an eighty-year-old woman who has been bed-bound for seven months due to weakness from gastric cancer. She has been married to eighty-six-year-old Gus for sixty-two years. During the past two years as Dolores's health issues intensified, Gus has been her main caregiver. Things have been rough for Dolores these last months. She often is in pain, has difficulty eating and drinking, and ruminates over the alienation she feels between herself and one of her three daughters.

When I raised the subject with Dolores about what helps her to cope, her eyes filled with tears. My initial reaction was to wonder: Is there nothing she feels that helps her? Did my question stir up feelings of despair and hopelessness? But my first impulse was wrong. Dolores pointed to Gus. Her gratitude for his love and care had triggered the flow of tearful emotion. With a wave-like gesture of her hand, she conveyed a desire to move onto another topic. "I'm going to cry if I start to talk about Gus."

I trust that many of us have experienced a scenario like the following. You walk into a house in which chaos and confusion is palpable. Everyone is rushing around, trying to tend to one crisis or another. And then you spot the elderly spouse of the patient, standing on the side, with a look of incomprehension on his or her face. You pause, look the individual in the eyes, and say with all the compassion you can muster, "How are *you* doing?" That's all it takes for the tears to flow. I would suggest that these are tears of gratitude, too—the gratitude a person feels in being noticed and attended to, of feeling worthy of another's compassion and concern.

We humans have a mixed relationship with tears. Sometimes we welcome them; other times we push them away. We may understand and accept how suffering induces tears, and how crying potentially can be cleansing and healing. I wonder, however, whether through welcoming and embracing the many flavors of tears, we can begin to make sense of and peace with a broader spectrum of life's most poignant moments.

I think of Jacob in the Bible. In his travels after his mother died, he came across the lovely Rachel, the woman who eventually would become his bride. In their encounter at the well, the text says, "Then Jacob kissed Rachel, and lifted up his voice and wept" (Gen 29:11). Tears of gratitude in finding love following a period of mourning were a salve for Jacob's grief. Years later, there is another mention of Jacob weeping, this time upon his reunification with his brother from whom he had long been separated after a bitter feud. The text says, "Then Esau ran to meet [Jacob] and embraced him, and fell on his neck and kissed him, and they wept" (Gen 34:4). These tears also reflect gratitude, in that reconciliation is possible even years after the bitterest of family feuds.

Whatever our relationship with tears, they potentially are a way to water our soul's capacity for growth; that is, when we meet them with kind curiosity, rather than judgment. While some tears give expression to our deepest sorrows, others deserve our attention as well. A line from the Psalms says, "Those who sow in tears shall reap in joy" (Ps 126:5).

When we meet tears with acceptance and patiently invite their exploration, when we honor all varieties of tears we might shed, life is fuller and richer. In giving today's tears their due, we prepare the ground for future growth, even perhaps for tomorrow's joy. In the midst of Dolores' pain, she rejoices in Gus's love for her.

May those who sow in tears reap in joy.

Contemplations

- What brings tears to my eyes?
- When are tears healing, and when not?
- How do I respond to others' tears?
- Is there anything I would change either about my own tears or about how I respond to others' tears?

An Affirmation for Me

When I meet my tears with acceptance and curiosity, I honor possibilities for the learning and growth that make life fuller and richer.

A Prayer to Share

They will come weeping, and with compassion will I guide them. Jer 31:9

> God, my tears are at the surface of my eyes,
> so often now, ready to flow,
> more easily than ever.

Primed to reveal my distress, confusion,
hopelessness, gratitude, uncertainty, anger.
A fountain of emotion.
Please help me God, to be curious,
to meet my tears with tenderness,
You, Who have received my tears
from childhood to the present day
with compassion.
When I come weeping,
You promise me consolation.
Open my eyes to see beyond my tears
to the joy of Your guidance
through life's overflow.

TONY: OUR WHOLE SELVES

Have you ever walked out of a visit feeling that it went well, but that to be effective you had to draw on every professional skill you have, all your life experience, and every ounce of your compassion? Have you ever said to yourself, *"This visit took everything I've got"*?

Tony is forty-two-years old, married with two young children. He was diagnosed a few months ago with ALS (amyotrophic lateral sclerosis). The disease is progressing quickly, with Tony already using a wheelchair and observing losses in his physical capacities daily. Tony, a competitive bowler, is nationally ranked. He owns a bowling alley and takes pride in his business skills. Besides concerns about his physical condition, he worries about finances. Throughout our visit, his forty-year-old wife Melinda was tearful. Tony acknowledged feeling waves of emotion, but his affect remained calm and controlled. Tony does not identify with any religion, claiming that spiritual pursuits have never been "his thing."

Why did this visit with Tony and Melinda require such an all-encompassing array of my professional skills and personal strengths? There is the obvious—assisting someone in exploring how best to cope with the enormity of a life-changing, cruel, and eventually fatal illness is a tremendous undertaking. There is also identifying and discussing issues specific to each individual patient dealing with such an overwhelming diagnosis.

For example, a specific theme in my conversation with Tony was about control. Tony sees his whole life up until his diagnosis as built on the gratification of being in control. Life had been meaningful because when he set his mind to something, he accomplished his goals, met his intentions. His success in bowling required him to cultivate a physical and mental tenacity that reliably demonstrated that you get what you want when you put in the effort. Through concentrated self-control, he would align the ball, his body, and his movements perfectly to achieve success. He also felt confident in his personal relationships, trusting in his well-calculated actions and behavior. Now, after the ALS diagnosis, Tony feels the need for a completely new infrastructure to anchor his sense of meaning. Being in control, as his operating life philosophy and source of gratification, isn't going to work for him anymore. Helping Tony to recreate his life philosophy and personal identity in ways that will feel trustworthy and meaningful, yet authentic to him, is no small task!

Another theme has to do with how to help Tony live in a now that feels bloated with the past and future. A familiar aspiration of spiritual life is to practice living in the present moment, as much as possible. With a diagnosis as dire as ALS, the past and the future can overwhelm the present. Focusing on how much better things were in the past and all the person has lost can crowd out the present from one direction. From the other direction, imagining the losses to come can be terrifying. When visiting Tony, my great challenge was to honor his losses and explore his fears, but also to assist him in finding ways that were authentic to him of experiencing peace in the present moment.

ALS, among other conditions we deal with, is a devastating diagnosis, raising questions such as: *Who am I now? What have I lost? Who can I be? What can I hope for in the future? How do I truly understand my place in my family and my place in the world? What are my values now and how might they need to change? Will it be possible for me ever to feel at peace?* To journey with others through what is a complete upheaval of the very foundation of their being likely will challenge us to draw on the fullness of *our own* professional knowledge, life experience, compassion, and spiritual identity—that is, everything we've got. I affirm that those in the healthcare world need to be mindful to avoid caregiver fatigue. At the same time, to be in this field, we understand that some situations will require us to step up. It's not always easy, but can there be a more sacred honor than the opportunity to step up with our whole selves?

Contemplations

- How do I understand my place in my family and my place in the world?
- What kinds of situations make it hard for me to step up?
- When stepping up is difficult, what strategies might I employ to help me identify hidden reserves of strength within myself?

An Affirmation for Me

Stepping up with our whole selves to be fully present to one who is hurting in body, mind, and spirit is to participate in a sacred journey.

A Prayer to Share

The Eternal God called out to the man, and said to him, "Where are you?" Gen 3:9

> I have so many questions these days,
> Questions it never occurred to me

That I would want to ask,
Would be in a situation
To feel compelled to ask.

Who am I now? What have I lost?
Who can I be? What can I hope for in the future?
How do I truly understand my place in my family and my place in the world?
What are my values now and how might they need to change?
Will it be possible for me to ever feel at peace?

So many questions for You, God;
For me; for us.
Yet, You have just one question for me:
"Where are you?"

Where am I, You ask?
I am here, at this moment,
Full of life.
I am with You.
And one day, when life leaves me,
Where will I be?
Still, with You.
God, You know where I am.
When I tune into the quiet of a day,
Listen into the pause that follows Your question,
I know the answer, too.
Where was I?
With You.
Where am I?
With You.
Where will I be?
With You.
Always with You.

PART 1: VIGNETTES

EDWIN: LOVING THE FACES OF GRIEF

How do you express love to those who need you when you yourself are deeply suffering? That was just one of the potent questions that arose in my mind working with Edwin.

The confluence of Edwin starting home care and his waking up to the truth of an unfathomable family tragedy drew the care team intensely into his life from the day he came onto service. Edwin, in his mid-sixties, began home care for wound management just five days after his twenty-seven-year-old son Barry, freakishly caught in the cross-fire of gang violence, was shot and killed. Barry had been the father of small children—four-year-old triplets and a new baby. Though he was young, Barry had been an independent, successful business owner. A family man, he had married his high school sweetheart Tiffany when they were both twenty years old. Edwin had been particularly close to his son Barry and his family, so close that with his declining health and limited finances, Edwin had recently accepted his son's invitation to move into the family's home.

Though there is much to contemplate around this staggering event, my comments focus on just one struggle: Edwin's angst around reaching out to his daughter-in-law Tiffany and the four grandchildren. Every day, Edwin would promise himself to call. The day would come, and the day would go. As much as he loved and deeply treasured Tiffany and the children, he just couldn't bring himself to dial the number. Even more daunting for him was imagining making the trip across town to the family's home to see the faces of these loved ones in person.

By my third visit with Edwin, I couldn't help but think of Tiffany. I imagined her wondering why she hadn't heard from her father-in-law after the funeral took place—now four weeks prior. How was she feeling—ignored, abandoned, hurt, angry? I projected how I might feel and what others have told me about how they've felt when those they love fail to be in touch when they are hurting terribly. I empathized with my "projected" Tiffany. Having sat with Edwin in his pain, having witnessed his emotional suffering, I couldn't blame Edwin either. Envisioning himself contacting them was torturing him, and *not* contacting them was torturing him too. Might he imagine that when he would see the faces of his grandchildren, as much as they are a source of joy and hope and blessing, they would remind him unbearably of the depth of his loss? In their young faces, he would see that of his now-deceased son. When I risked sharing this possibility, Edwin dropped his head into his hands. It seemed I had touched upon his fears. After a few moments of silence, he raised his head. "Tomorrow," he said, "I'm going to visit tomorrow."

I realized in reflecting on this situation how easy it is, when we feel someone we love has let us down, to picture that person as heartless, thoughtless, inconsiderate, or worse. Sitting with Edwin was a profound reminder of the complexity of sorrow and suffering and the futility of blaming. Regardless of how Tiffany felt, I saw how lost and broken Edwin was. You never can know what others are experiencing, the depths of their sorrows. You never know how others may wish to be more or to do more than they feel they can. It's far too easy for feelings of grief to be displaced by other, seemingly "safe" emotions. Blame may step in for grief when grief becomes too much to bear. Author and speaker Brené Brown, PhD, says, "Blame is the discharging of discomfort and pain."[1] Whether dealing with our patients' grief or our own, we will be at our wisest and most compassionate when we notice, recognize, and appreciate the power of grief.

Contemplations

- What are my biggest challenges around judgment of others?
- When has there been a time when my being judgmental got in the way of my compassion?
- How do I stay as attentive as possible to resisting blame?
- What are the most healthful ways for me to discharge discomfort and pain?

1. "Brown, "Brené Brown on Blame."

Part 1: Vignettes

An Affirmation for Me

The humility to admit that I can never know for certain what others are experiencing guides me to be patient, kind, and compassionate.

A Prayer to Share

Do not hide from me; do not reject Your servant. You have always been my help; do not abandon me. Forsake me not, O God, my deliverer. Ps 27:9

> I want to do the right thing,
> but doing so takes energy, motivation, and courage—
> and I am so depleted.
> Where will I find the strength
> to reach out to those who may count on me,
> or to reach inward to attend to the intensity of my own suffering?
> There are moments when I not only want to hide from others,
> but from myself, as well.
> To sleep for hours on end. Make the pain go away.
> But for the moment, I am awake,
> and so entrust my lack of will to You, God.
> The reality of this day,
> the burdens of my sorrows
> I hand over to You.
> In surrendering,
> I invite Your presence to sustain me,
> to give me courage.
> Since I know You believe in me,
> and that I can do the right thing,
> I will be able to do so.

III.

Attending to Fear

FEAR CAN INTERRUPT, SLOW down, diminish, or even paralyze the healing process. In the next four vignettes, fear emerges as a great hurdle for progressing toward improving physical, emotional, relational, and/or spiritual well-being. Strangely, if we were to encapsulate what are the two most common fears, we could suggest they are opposites. On one hand, there is fear of the unknown, and on the other, fear of the known, that is, of the (presumably) known unpleasant, difficult, painful, or frightening. (On one hand: "I don't know what will show up on the MRI, and therefore am fearful." On the other hand: "I once had an MRI, and because it was frightening then, I am fearful now in anticipating it.") A parallel pair of opposites is: the fear of change versus the fear of no change.

The stories that follow explore fears that fall onto one side of these polarities or the other, or even shift back and forth. As caregivers, we cannot cure another person of his or her fear. Our empathy, patience, and integrity, however, may make just the difference in supporting another to begin to release his or her fear, or at least to live with more peace and self-acceptance with regard to this difficult emotion.

Part 1: Vignettes

KAY: A VISION OF EXPANSIVENESS

Kay was on home care recovering from shoulder surgery. After a few weeks, this former hospice nurse came down with a cough that, to her shock, turned out to be an aggressive lung cancer. The originating source of the cancer was still unknown by the time she was discharged from home care. Kay's hunch was that she would die within a year.

In my last visit, she was anticipating an MRI, a prospect that frightened her terribly. She was afraid of the confinement, the claustrophobia she expected with the test. "Could you come up with a short prayer I could say while I'm in that machine?" she asked me. While she did not practice a specific religion, she had a sense of the sacred and even had become tearful when I gave her a blessing on a previous visit. A verse from Psalms came to mind as a fitting "MRI" prayer. I offered her these words from Psalm 118:5, and they deeply touched and comforted her: "From the Narrow place I called out to God, who answered me with the Divine Expanse."

Whether or not you come from a tradition that embraces a faith in God, there's an underlying wisdom in the psalm that can speak to most patients and even to ourselves as care providers; that is, we all find ourselves in "narrow places"—places of fear, of constriction. It is in those times when our world feels small and constraining that we experience our worries and troubles as confining us, beating us down.

The challenge becomes to step back, to get perspective, to see a bigger picture, to connect to something beyond our pain. Some people connect with the idea of trust in God's expansiveness. For others, the connection to the bigger picture is through a focus on family or pets, activities, or specific values. One thing we can do as care providers is to encourage those for whom we care—especially when they are fearful and despairing—to connect with those things, those people, those experiences that breathe expansiveness into their lives.

Contemplations

- What are some of the narrow places I've encountered in my own life?
- Among those for whom I've cared, what are some of the most difficult narrow places they have had to navigate?
- What words would I use for others or for myself when they or I become fearful—whether it be of an MRI machine or of some other narrow place, physical or psychological?

An Affirmation for Me

When navigating narrow places or figuratively negotiating narrow ideas and perspectives, I manage fear by connecting with those things, people, and experiences that breathe expansiveness into my life.

A Prayer to Share

From the Narrow place I called out to God, who answered me with the Divine Expanse. Psalm 118:5

> Infinite God,
> You have no beginning and no end;
> Eternal and forever,
> You enlighten me with Your vastness—
> The sky beyond the clouds affirms how
> Your constant Presence pervades.
> Help me to breathe Your expansiveness
> Into all the tight, tense, tangled, and taut
> Places within me.

PART 1: VIGNETTES

> In my crying and calling out to you,
> I release myself into Your Spirit.
> Since You are forever,
> I forever travel with You.

DORA: POWERLESSNESS

One of the most heartbreaking situations we come across in home care visits is to interact with weakened and vulnerable patients who are dependent on someone, usually a family member, who does not treat them well. One patient who breaks my heart is fifty-six-year-old Dora who has been coping with multiple ailments that have left her homebound for several years. In addition to dealing with the challenges of managing chronic pain and the need for intravenous feedings, Dora is prone to infections and pneumonia. Her husband Evan, for the most part, gets her to medical appointments, runs household errands, and assists her physically when she has difficulty ambulating. However, he can be cold, visibly resentful, and cruel in the way he speaks to her, as well as delayed in his responsiveness to her needs.

Due to complex dynamics in the marriage, unstable finances, alienation from extended family members, and general social isolation, Dora feels she has no choice but to depend on Evan who does provide her with the basic care she needs. Dora insists she is getting by adequately enough and that intervention by Adult Protective Services would be an overreaction. After conferring with the social worker who had visited this home on numerous occasions, I also agreed that alerting Adult Protective Services was not the route to go at this time, even though there are circumstances in which a patient is being abused, and this must be reported, even against a patient's wishes.

In my visits with Dora, she shares her worries and disappointments, as well as her hopes. Reflecting on memories of better times helps give her strength. Prayer and her religious faith are integral to her daily coping. Her two cats delight her with their loving companionship. Although I am encouraged that Dora has some reliable coping strategies, mostly I feel powerless. Her underlying circumstances are of deep concern with each day a struggle. Being dependent on Evan exacerbates the struggle. While Dora remains in an unhealthy relationship, she is adamant about preserving the status quo.

Our role as care providers focuses on listening, assessing, and implementing healing interventions. We can share our observations with patients, encourage them to consider making changes, and educate them about options. Ultimately, however, patients make their own choices about how they will live. I know I'm not alone in feeling powerless in certain situations we encounter in home care. On one hand, we know we have to accept our limitations with regard to eliminating others' suffering. On the other, as healers and problem solvers, surrendering to limitations and admitting to feelings of powerlessness is not easy.

Our hearts may break for those who are dependent on others who are unkind to them. My intention and belief is that by giving my full attention to these vulnerable patients and treating them with dignity, kindness, and patience, I offer an alternate experience, a touchstone for reassurance. When I am not there and Dora is enduring a difficult interchange with Evan, my hope is that somewhere deep inside her, that memory of being treated well and feeling worthy of kindness will help ease Dora's present moment struggle, even for the tiniest bit. I am not able to alleviate all Dora is facing, but I trust that the difference that even a few moments of kindness make is worthwhile. Such moments can be a foundation for her to face her challenges with more peace and equanimity.

It can be difficult to rise above those waves of powerlessness that come upon us in our work with patients. But I believe one of the antidotes is to trust that something does shift for the better in our patients when we show up and persist in expressing, embodying, and modeling kindness.

Contemplations

- What caregiving situation(s) make me feel powerless?
- How have I dealt with a situation in which my own hopes for the patient/family clashed with their goals? . . . Would there be a better way?
- How do I cope with feelings of powerlessness?

An Affirmation for Me

When I feel powerless, I remind myself that I can't control choices others make—sometimes all I can do is to remain kind, even when I don't agree.

A Prayer to Share

"Not by might nor by power, but by my Spirit," says the Eternal God Almighty. Zech 4:5

> God, how shall I act,
> What shall I do—
> When my body is depleted,
> My concentration sapped,
> And my motivation dwindles precariously?
> With moving being difficult, and becoming still,
> Harder yet,
> I feel powerless.
>
> But what is power anyway?
> An illusion.
> Everything that was once mighty,
> Eventually weakens—
> The body ages,

The roof needs repair,
Potholes appear on the streets,
Communities must reinvent themselves,
Crops need rotation,
Hillsides erode.

But You are the Eternal God.
When all else fades, diminishes, or disappears,
You remain,
Your Spirit suffusing all things.
You were, You are, You will be—
Past, present, and future.
Releasing my life into Your hands,
I am fortified—
Your Spirit is in me always.

DANA CUDDLED

One of my patients, seventy-year-old Dana is often anxious and scared. In my efforts to help her, I asked if there were any pleasant memories that she could go to in her mind that might provide comfort and reassurance. Although typically filled with agitation and wracked with worry, Dana replied that there is one image she returns to time and again, day and night, that offers her some relief. As I sat with her, she described how when she was little and couldn't sleep, she would tiptoe into her parents' bedroom. She would climb into their bed—her father on one side, her mother next to him. As Dana scooted in, her mother would wrap her arms around her, enveloping Dana within the curve of her body. In my hour-long visit with Dana, this image was the one comfort we could identify as helping soothe her angst and hopelessness.

What a powerful image! In home care we hear so much about patients' fears, disappointments, and worries—all the things they expect to cause problems and, too often, do. What is easy to forget is that as much as humans may be vulnerable to problems, the capacity for inner peace is every bit as much a part of our humanity. Illness will intrude upon most all of our life stories. Even as illness may be inseparable from the human story, however, so too is the possibility for inner peace.

Most of us have a time, a place, or a moment in which we felt safe, when we felt embraced and cared for. What is that place? When was that moment? How did it feel? What did we see, taste, smell, and hear? This memory balm is an ally of hope. As surely as our patients may need prescribed medications, they also need hope. They need touchstones, memories, possibilities, and reassurances that something greater than their current pain can hold them, keep them safe, soften their fears. Some patients, such as Dana, may surrender fear to the felt memory of a mother's embrace. For others, it is their faith that they are held by God that sustains them. Still for others, their spirits may be lifted by the memory of moments in which they met life with wholeheartedness and gratitude. We can encourage those we serve to allow themselves to bask in the healing properties of those feelings, memories, thoughts, and prayers that give them hope, courage, and the faith that their lives matter.

Contemplations

- When and where have I felt safe?
- What was that experience like—what did I see, taste, smell, and hear?
- What one image might especially capture that feeling?
- What do I notice in my body, mind, and heart if I spend a few moments closing my eyes and focusing on that image?
- When might it be most helpful for me to remember to return to this image as a source of calm and reassurance?

An Affirmation for Me

My calm and reassuring presence with patients offers a welcome refuge, inviting feelings of safety and security.

A Prayer to Share

I will dwell in Your tent forever; I will take refuge beneath the shelter of Your wings. Ps 61:4

> God, it's hard sometimes to stay connected to You.
> I can feel agitated, angry, confused, and frustrated
> by everything I have to cope with.
> So often, I'm in pain—
> whether I feel it in my body, or in my relationships,
> or due to the many often overwhelming practical matters I have to keep track of.
> I wish I could just cuddle up with someone I love
> and forget all my troubles.
> In my life there have been moments of loving cuddling,
> and moments when I have felt the dearth of that feeling of safety and security.
> Help me to remember, God,
> that You are my ever-present Loving Companion,
> and that Your warm expansiveness
> invites me to take refuge in You.
> You are there to embrace me in the shelter of Your wings.
> Please embrace me now. I need You. I am Yours. With You, I am safe.

Part 1: Vignettes

POLLY: FEAR'S RANGE OF MOTION

How can we help patients navigate their fears? Polly is a sixty-two-year-old woman who is suffering from interrelated ailments related to falls, back pain, a neuromuscular disorder, wounds from a broken leg, and obesity. She lives alone in a small, tidy home in a friendly neighborhood. Polly feels stuck—not only with regard to her physical condition, but in many other dimensions of her life as well. Though she is coping with many stressors, the spiritual stress that stands out above the rest is fear.

Polly needs another surgery. She is both afraid and afraid not to have the surgery. In dealing with insurance company hassles, she fears she may not get all the interventions that would most benefit her. She is isolated and knows she needs more help, but fears introducing a stranger into her home. Her walker was damaged in her last fall. While she hopes to get a new one soon, finances are tight. She fears using the damaged walker, but also fears not using it at all. She is well aware that her weight exacerbates her medical concerns, but it has become too difficult to get out to attend her weight-management support group. She fears she may never be able to surmount this lifelong problem.

Fear can be debilitating. In the face of intense fear, our sympathetic nervous system kicks in, compelling us to fight the fear, flee from it, or freeze in our tracks. The hormonal cascade that comes with these responses can antagonize the healing process. As healers, we may need to help our patients with their fears. One thing humans fear most is the unknown. Figuring out exactly what our patients are most afraid of may help. Humans also fear change. Clarifying with patients the potential benefits of a proposed change may make the change more bearable.

At times, I imagine most health caregivers become stymied by our patients' fears. How do we adequately address the fears patients experience as so enormous and intransigent? How do we help someone who is afraid to do something, but afraid not to; afraid to take a medication, but afraid not to; afraid to get caregiver help, but afraid not to; afraid to communicate openly with a loved one, but afraid not to; perhaps afraid even to live, but afraid to die?

In addressing Polly's fear to bring help into her home, she and I made a list of all her questions and concerns. Seeing the chaos of her worries contained on a paper, helped alleviate both Polly's fear of the unknown as well as her fear of change. The list also would aid her in discussing her needs with a caregiver agency. Although Polly's past experience with meditation suggested that this tool could help ease her anxiety, she had become fearful that she would just get settled and calm in her meditation when a surge of pain would jar her. We discussed how, rather than going to a place of annoyance with herself for getting distracted, she could respond to her pain by saying to herself, "May I be free from suffering," and then gently return her attention back to her meditation. Having Polly write down her worries and use kinder self-talk are small, simple examples of interventions to help Polly with her fear.

Healthcare clinicians are familiar with how small, simple steps can contribute significantly to patients' physical well-being. I suggest drawing on a range-of-motion metaphor, expanding its application to emotional, interpersonal, spiritual, and adherence-to-care-plan challenges. For example, when a person first comes home from the hospital after shoulder surgery, the therapist expects minimal movement, but gradually, in small, incremental stages, range of motion expands.

Those we serve are often as emotionally and spiritually vulnerable as they are physically vulnerable. Goals on all of these levels may need to start small. With gentleness, persistence, and patience many, if not most, of our patients can achieve a greater emotional and spiritual range of motion. I have witnessed how steadfast and patient home care clinicians with whom I work remain when patients' physical healing progresses slowly. Can we remain as steadfast and patient with the healing of minds and hearts? Can we be as steadfast and patient with the slow, painful process of a woman like Polly expanding her range of motion by learning to slowly release her tight grip on fear?

Part 1: Vignettes

Contemplations

- What do I fear?
- What helps allay my fears?
- What do my patients/those for whom I care fear?
- What would be three incremental steps I might practice myself and suggest to my patients for addressing fear (or another difficult emotion, such as, worry, anger, or hopelessness)?

An Affirmation for Me

Knowing that true healing requires investment of the whole self, I maintain as steadfast a commitment to the healing of patients' minds and hearts, as to their bodies,

A Prayer to Share

Do not fear, for I am with you; do not be dismayed, for I am your God. I will strengthen you and help you; I will uphold you with my righteous right hand. Isa 41:10

> God, this fear! Why does it feel so insistent, so tenacious?
> In dismay I turn to You,
> To Your promise of reassurance—
> Your promise to uphold, strengthen, and simply be with me.
> And yet,
> I drift from You—
> A moment here and a moment there—
> Away from reassurance, and back to fear.
> I remember how You hold me up, and then I forget.
> I relax into Your embrace, and later become numb to it.
> I step toward You, and slip back.
> But even if I forget, become numb, or slip,

Attending to Fear

You always are stepping toward me.
Help me to find the courage to persist—
Each step toward You,
Small as it may be,
Is a step closer to Your peace,
To Your calm, and to the hope of new possibilities.
Wherever I am,
You meet me and draw me near,
You whisper to me, saying—
"Lean on Me more confidently,
Trust in yourself more freely,
My help and My strength are as close as
your next step, your next breath."

IV.

Overcoming Challenges to Connecting

Entering into a new caregiving situation means encountering many unknowns. We may feel an instant connection with someone, or it may take days, weeks, or months for a meaningful bond to develop. Then there are situations in which a sense of disconnection pervades and persists. The challenge for caregivers is to continue to go toward the discomfort rather than away—to be with it, learn about it, negotiate with it, and maybe someday even befriend it. There are those cases in which we may need to bow out, for one of a range of reasons, such as removing ourselves from a dangerous environment. But when the situation does not disintegrate into the rare exception that calls for more extreme responses, we may find we learn and grow the most through those moments of discomfort and from our reflections on the disconnects.

JOSEPH AND ADELE: WHAT IS YOUR PRODUCT? WHY ARE YOU HERE?

I visited eighty-five-year-old Joseph in his modest, cluttered, but well-kept home. He seemed pleased to have me visit and, almost immediately, launched into his theory of different religions. Using the image of two airplanes representing different companies flying to the same destination, he made this analogy: "When two hearts are joined, different religions don't matter." After about twenty minutes of elaboration on his spiritually universalistic worldview, he paused and looked at me. "So what is your product?" he asked.

My product? Though I was a bit puzzled by this phraseology, I responded by naming various ways chaplains may provide support—through assisting in exploring coping strategies, offering encouragement, normalizing feelings, affirming strengths, helping patients find resources for meaning and hope or for dealing with grief... and for some sharing prayer or reading Scriptures. Recognizing the need to move beyond an academic explanation, I shifted to focusing on what I heard in his story, how I was touched by his compassion, courage, and the open-heartedness of his words.

After the visit with Joseph, I headed over to the home of Adele, an 85-year-old woman recuperating from a fall who had some short-term memory loss. Adele's granddaughter, Beth, as well as Adele's caregiver, were present. When Adele asked me, "Why are you here?" I started to explain when Beth piped in, reminding Adele how connected she had been to her Catholicism, how precious her religious practice and heritage were to her, and how Beth thought the chaplain would be a welcome visitor. Adele did not seem terribly convinced, but we carried on with the visit. Shortly after Beth left, Adele asked me again, "Why are you here?" Now it was the caregiver and myself offering explanations, describing the role of the chaplain, what I could offer, and so on. Again, Adele seemed lukewarm, but we continued in conversation, until the next time: "Why are you here?" By the fourth or fifth repetition of this question, the caregiver and I looked at each other and shrugged in nonverbal agreement to keep it simple. "I'm here to spend some time with you," I responded with a smile. Later, as I was leaving, Adele thanked me and said, "Nice of you to take the time to visit the old folks."

What is your product? Why are you here? It is true that we may need to clarify to our patients the basics of what our roles are as home care professionals. On one hand, while we may accept the necessity of responding succinctly and articulately to such questions, we may consider them to be routine and elementary. On the other hand, the questions—"What do you have to offer?" and "Why are you here?"—touch on foundational spiritual, existential considerations. Our responses reflect our essential motivations for living and being. Hard to get more profound than that!

Interestingly, the first question God asks a human being in the Bible is, "Where are you?" This is when God addresses Adam after he and Eve have eaten the forbidden fruit, and Adam attempts to hide from God . . . as if anyone actually *can* hide from God. The question "Where are you?" is probably not a location clarification. Rather God challenges Adam/man to consider something deeper about the essence and purpose of his existence. The last question chronologically in the Hebrew Bible that God addresses to a human being is to Elijah. God asks: "What are you doing here?" The bookends of the Hebrew Bible present questions not so different from the questions Joseph and Adele had for me. You probably have received similar ones.

If we live an attentive, conscientious life, we will wrestle with profound spiritual questions, such as: "What is your product?" "Why are you here?" "Where are you?" "What are you doing here?" Our responses may vary, given different contexts and seasons in our own lives. However, when all is said and done and we simplify the complex explanations for our patients, we may find ourselves conveying something as streamlined as what I said to Adele: "I'm here to spend some time with you." In our hearts, we silently may feel inspired by the words of Ram Dass: "We're all just walking each other home."[1]

---

1. Crumm, "The Ram Dass interview: Smiling as he teaches about 'Polishing the Mirror.'"

Contemplations

- What is your "product?" In other words, What do you offer others? What do you offer the world?
- Why are you here?
- Where are you spiritually?

An Affirmation for Me

In being someone who listens, cares, and heals, I am a blessing.

A Prayer to Share

"What are you doing here, Elijah? . . . What are you doing here, Elijah?" I Kgs 19:9 and 19:13

> God, I wonder why I am here—
> Is there a plan for me;
> Something You want me to accomplish;
> A reason for my being,
> For awakening to a new day?
>
> Divine Light, remind me to see each moment
> As an opportunity for kindness;
> Each encounter
> As an invitation for expressing encouragement,
> gratitude, affirmation.
> Bless me with the knowledge
> That each day is a palette
> With infinite possibilities
> For extending blessing and
> For recreating myself as a blessing.
> I am here to embody
> Your blessings.

Part 1: Vignettes

GRACIA: LANGUAGE OF THE HEART

On my second visit to 87-year-old Gracia, her son Pedro was also present. Gracia sat in her wheelchair, and Pedro sat on Gracia's bed. I pulled up a chair. Gracia and Pedro were finishing up a conversation about her eyeglasses. He said to her, "*La receta para tus anteojos debe ser correcta, pero si hay un problema,* we can take them back to the eyeglasses store."

The literal translation into English of what Pedro said to his mother was, "The prescription for your glasses should be correct, but if there's a problem, we can take them back to the eyeglasses store." Though my Spanish is far from 100 percent, I got the gist of the half-Spanish, half-English sentence. Both Gracia and her son are native English speakers, but with their bilingual facility, they shifted from one language to the other as they finished discussing a few practical matters before Pedro left Gracia and me to continue our own conversation.

It's one thing to catch only part of what might be the literal translation of words in a foreign language, but what I found with Gracia was that the subtleties of understanding her were more complex. Because of her way of verbalizing, more than half of her words sounded garbled to me. Even so, I grasped most of what she expressed.

There are times when a clinician may need to be persistent in understanding a patient's exact words, such as when he or she describes symptoms of an illness. However, in my listening to Gracia freely sharing from her heart, I felt it would detract from our rapport to ask her continually to repeat herself. She told me about her relationships with family members, recalled memories of her deceased husband and international travels, spoke about the importance of prayer for coping with her sadness and anxiety, and more. Somehow, although I comprehended a low percentage of her specific words, I was able to respond and empathize such that she felt encouraged to keep sharing in ways that released many pent-up emotions.

On one hand, I wondered whether there is something deceitful about "playing along," implying that I'm understanding everything when I'm not. On the other hand, I felt I *did understand*. Moreover, my compassion was 100 percent authentic. With some research, I came across studies indicating that between 70 and 90 percent of all communication is nonverbal. Thus, it is not just a poetic expression to say that two individuals can communicate "heart to heart." In fact, it may be that most of what we communicate *is* heart to heart, as well as eye to eye, gesture to gesture, facial expression to facial expression . . . more so than word to word. Words have their place, but other significant ways of knowing and becoming known to another are equally, if not more, potent.

Philosopher Martin Buber wrote about three spheres of relating: with nature, with another person, or with a spiritual being. In each, we may encounter the other fully with our whole being in what Buber names an "I-and-Thou" relationship. With regard to the spiritual sphere of relating, Buber says, "Here the relation is wrapped in a cloud, but reveals itself." Even without words, a certain language of connectedness can emerge. Thus, in a human-to-human "I-and-Thou" relationship, we may gaze "toward the fringe of the eternal *Thou* . . . in each *Thou* we address the eternal *Thou*."

There are patients, like Gracia, with whom the communication cannot rely completely on words. Through a heart-to-heart encounter, we may sense ourselves glimpsing beyond the parameters of the immediate interchange to gaze into the realm of the eternal *Thou,* into the sphere of the holy.

Contemplations

- How aware am I of my body language?
- Have I ever gotten feedback about my body language that caught me by surprise? If so, what was the feedback, and what have I learned from it?
- How aware am I of others' body language?
- In reflecting on an important "heart-to-heart" encounter from my life, what qualities were present?

Part 1: Vignettes

An Affirmation for Me

I cultivate awareness of my tone of voice, the quality of my gaze, and how tense or calm I am in my body, in order to maximize and reinforce my intention to be fully present to those for whom I care.

A Prayer to Share

Moses said to God, "Pardon Your servant, God. I have never been a man of words, either in times past or now that You have spoken to Your servant. I am slow of speech and slow of tongue." Exod 4:10

God, You know every thought in my mind,
Every feeling in my heart,
Every ache in my body.
But when my thoughts and feelings
become garbled or confused,
words escape me,
Sometimes, not budging at all—
refusing the trip from head to lips.

I'm often slow now—
Can't think of what to say, how to say it,
Can't locate precise vocabulary to convey
Swirling torrents within me.
Yet I take comfort in that—

You know every thought in my mind,
Every feeling in my heart,
Every ache in my body.
I entrust my soul and spirit to Your ever-present,
Quiet love.

Overcoming Challenges to Connecting

PHYLLIS: AMBIGUITY OF OUTCOMES

The attendees at the case conference consulted grimly. How to keep sixty-eight-year-old Phyllis from landing on the streets felt nearly impossible. Yet, we clung to the notion of "nearly." "Nearly impossible" didn't mean there wasn't some way to find a new home for her. Phyllis has cognitive challenges and is partially deaf. She was on home care for a skin infection. Her sister, with whom she was living in an SRO (single-resident-occupancy) hotel, had died the week before. Phyllis's grief engulfed her. On a practical level, she was also overwhelmed. She didn't have sufficient income to continue to pay for the small room she and her sister had shared for the last eleven years. Phyllis had no other family and no friends. The only people taking an interest in her life were the home care staff.

Our home care team mobilized on all fronts. There had to be a way to avoid a rapidly encroaching tragedy. The social worker reached out to every organization, agency, board and care (group home), and social services consultant she could think of. Our home care director connected with his contacts in the broader hospital system for their input. Other clinicians on the care team buoyed Phyllis' spirits and hopes as she waited for updates as to where she might be able to move. After many hours of intensive, extensive efforts, a board and care was found that would accept Phyllis as a resident, even with her limited means to pay. This particular board and care is in a rural part of the county, with lovely woods surrounding the property. There are beautiful flower and vegetable gardens around the home, and a tranquil feeling pervades. The home itself is spacious, nicely furnished, clean, and comfortable. When our social worker enthusiastically shared with the team her success in placing Phyllis, I was excited to visit. The efforts had paid off! Phyllis would be well cared for and safe.

When I arrived at Phyllis's new home, I found her in her bedroom. Within moments, she teared up. She felt trapped, stuck. She felt disconnected from the other residents, all of whom were older than she. She considered the meal times to be overly rigid. There was nowhere to walk—no shops or restaurants or parks, no pets. It was all so confining. She couldn't imagine living here for what could be twenty or more years! Phyllis felt ashamed about her complaints, but couldn't help airing them. I did my best to listen, empathize, reframe, and encourage her to explore strategies for feeling better about the situation. I felt sad and discouraged, too, that Phyllis was feeling so down.

Shortly after her move, Phyllis was discharged from our care. Presumably she continues to adjust. She may be happier than when I saw her, or she may not. Though on a practical level Phyllis' desperate living circumstances were reversed, we couldn't help but hope that Phyllis would be appreciative, that she would rejoice in having been given a new home, a new community, natural beauty, safety, and comfort. How do we process such a situation? We did the best we could. We were confident that we had pursued and succeeded in attaining the optimal outcome. We honored the patient's needs and preferences as much as possible given constrictive variables beyond our control. Yet, the message that comes back to us is that the person we thought we had helped is disappointed, dissatisfied, and unhappy.

A spiritual teaching that I find especially relevant to such scenarios has its roots in the Hindu sacred text, the *Bhagavad Gita*. The text advises renouncing the fruit of our actions. That means that at any given moment we do what we believe is the right thing, the best thing. We do so lovingly, selflessly, and as skillfully as possible, and then we renounce any concern for the result. The text says, "The awakened sages call a person wise when all their undertakings are free from anxiety about results" (3:19). A specific practice I came across suggests, "Upon arising in the morning, and at night before falling asleep, or any time you feel relaxed, make a mental suggestion to your mind that whatever you do in the coming day, you will release the fruits, and perform all acts simply because they are right and virtuous and appropriate for you to do—regardless of whether they turn out the way you think they should."[2]

---

2. Nitya, "Living Your Practice: Meditation in Action," 102.

Contemplations

- What patient care situations particularly bother me, even when I may know rationally that they involve variables beyond my control?
- How do I respond when what I feel is the very best I have to offer does not meet others' hopes and expectations?
- What are healthy ways for me to respond to disappointments—whether others' disappointments in me or my disappointments in myself?

An Affirmation for Me

When I do what I believe is right and kind, I can let go of judging myself on outcomes, as they are beyond my control.

A Prayer to Share

"For I know the plans I have for you," declares the Eternal, plans for peace and not for harm, plans to give you a hopeful future. Jer 29:11

> God, I feel trapped, stuck.
> There are those who try to help me,
> but still I feel disappointed.
> Life has not turned out the way I had hoped.
> In fact, day by day, life feels more dreary.
> The support I get is not enough to sweeten the bitterness
> that greets me when I wake up, and that stubbornly clings to me
> throughout my difficult days.
> I may be stubborn, too, but why should I settle for
> what feels to me like a compromised life?
> I long for joy, for enthusiasm, for freedom.

Part 1: Vignettes

> You, who are the Source of peace,
> Whose plan for me is peace,
> Please show me a way to peace.
> Even through the disappointments,
> I trust there are opportunities for respite.
> Help me to see beauty I may have overlooked,
> Kindnesses I may not have appreciated,
> Quiet moments of reassuring calm.
> Open me to noticing sparks of Your promise,
> Sparks of the hopeful future You
> Have in store for me.

MARLA AND DON: SURPRISE TWISTS AND TURNS

This vignette is similar to the previous one, although this time it was a family member who did *not* appreciate what I had to offer, and it didn't feel good!

Marla and Don, a couple in their sixties, married forty years, have grown children and several grandchildren. Marla's illness has consumed a good deal of the couple's resources. Despite the challenges, their faith helps keep them buoyed. Over the course of several visits, Marla and I had engaged in rich conversations—talking about the challenges of her illness, the centrality of her spiritual faith, and stories of her family. On my fourth visit, Marla's husband Don had some questions for me. He objected to the chaplain's commitment to honor and address each patient's personal religious (or no religion) preferences. Don's challenge was that I was *not* advocating for what *he* asserted to be the one true faith.

Don and I went back and forth—between my explanations of what an interfaith chaplain is and his insistence that my approach was "fluff." Marla patiently listened as Don and my conversation unfolded. Eventually it became clear to him that there were certain professional parameters that I would uphold—that my commitment is to respect and address each patient's *own* spiritual path.

After my engagement with Don wound down, he went back to his own tasks, turning the visit back over to Marla and me. Where did all of this leave her? She expressed that she enjoyed and appreciated our visits, found them helpful, and would like to continue. I have made three visits since then. Marla continues to benefit from our interactions, and Don continues to voice his challenging opinions.

It's probably natural to feel thrown off when a patient or family member gets disparagingly confrontational. I know that has been my experience. How to handle confrontation is a whole topic in and of itself, so I'll mention just one often overlooked but vital consideration: Remembering to be kind to ourselves. Even if there *is* something that we need to correct with regard to a specific situation, beating ourselves up does no one any good. After we take those few deep breaths when we are caught by surprise, we can remind ourselves that even if we have things to learn, ways to improve (and who doesn't?), we also have much wisdom to share. If we didn't, we wouldn't be doing this job. We also have resources and consultants to support us. Even if a patient or family member's outburst stems from an *unsupported* concern, it still can sting. Kindness to ourselves will help us get through and make the best decisions moving forward.

As the Buddhist teacher Jack Kornfeld so wisely instructs, *"If your compassion does not include yourself, it is incomplete."*[3]

Contemplations

- When have I experienced confrontation with someone I've cared for, and how did I handle the situation?
- What are my strategies for managing my own emotions during moments of confrontation?
- How am I wise?

---

3. Kornfeld, *Buddha's Little Instruction Book*, 28.

Part 1: Vignettes

An Affirmation for Me

When confrontation catches me by surprise, I remind myself that while everyone, including me, has things to learn, I also have much wisdom which, along with kindness to myself, will allow me to make the best decisions moving forward.

A Prayer to Share

For the sake of my family and friends, I will say, "Peace be within you." For the sake of the House of the Eternal God, I will seek your good. Ps 122:8–9

> God, among Your many names,
> You are called Peace.
> You, who are the canopy of
> Well-being, serenity, and equanimity,
> Beam toward me and through me
> Your warm rays of calm and clarity.
> You fill me with Your light,
> From my toes, through my legs,
> Up through my waist, hips, torso, and chest;
> From the tips of my fingers, through my hands and arms;
> Shoulders, neck, face, and to the top of my skull.
> I breathe, knowing I am complete.
> Your assurance streams through me, and
> I relax, knowing I am whole.
>
> Grant me peace—
> Peace within myself,
> Peace in my relationships,
> Peace with You.
> Thus, You prepare me to seek out
> The good in all creatures and all creation.

Overcoming Challenges to Connecting

Your peace and Your goodness
Become my peace and my goodness—
Ever expanding.
I thank You.

V.

Navigating Changes, Boundaries, and Borderlines

MEDICAL LINGO USES THE term *titration* to describe the process of determining the needed medication dosage to maximize symptom relief, while avoiding negative side effects. For example, a person at the end of life may take a dosage of morphine that would overwhelm and possibly kill a healthy individual. When a doctor has prescribed morphine in gradually stepped-up doses to keep up with a dying person's pain, the titration process is geared to provide appropriate and effective relief.

Similar to the art of prescribing medications, emotional and spiritual support can involve *titration;* that is, we continually assess when to "step-up" our engagement with a patient and when to hold steady and not push. There is no magic formula. The key is to be acutely attentive to each individual's unique capacities and unique circumstances. This means frequently asking ourselves and evaluating: When do I introduce a new thought, a new consideration, or a new approach? When is it best to allow for a period of adjustment, acclimatization, and status quo? Often, it is wise to start with small new considerations rather than all at once with a bold, and possibly overwhelming, whole new approach.

CINDY: PERMEABLE BOUNDARIES

My visits to fifty-eight-year-old Cindy take me to places beyond my familiar boundaries. One is to the dilapidated, trailer park, single-room home in which she resides, and a place her homeless friends drop in and out of. In my life, I've taken the walls of a home and a roof overhead for granted—as "boundaries" protecting me from the unpredictable elements of the outdoors. Another "place" beyond familiar boundaries is to a mind vulnerable to unwelcome voices. Cindy has schizophrenia and often hears voices, like trespassers, who threaten her ability to see herself as an autonomous, reliably consistent, recognizable self. In my life, I take the boundaries of my mind for granted. Though my thoughts and feelings can shift moment to moment, I experience them as authentically expressing only my own voice.

Stale smoke air in the room we sit in adds to the sense of ambiguous boundaries. Cindy claims to have given up smoking three years ago. The room is not blatantly smoky, but the air is not clear either. She shares stories of individuals who communicate with her from her television. At the same time, she conveys that she understands these relationships are not real. She speaks of various friends who stay in her home. To the degree that this may or may not be factual is not my concern as much as whether she is comfortable and feels safe with these visitors. Her comments assert that she does feel comfortable and safe. As I listen with respect and without judgment, I affirm the insights she expresses about her physical and mental coping. It seems she feels comfortable and safe with me. Although her assessment of reality does not always mesh with my own, we have developed a rapport, and she freely shares details of her daily life, along with reflections on what gives her life meaning.

In our healthcare world, we talk about the importance of maintaining professional boundaries. Guidelines may address appropriate boundaries in the realms of emotions, finances, physical contact, personal self-disclosure, and so on. Boundaries come up in the spiritual world too. There are prayers in my faith tradition that reflect an appreciation for the distinction between the sacred and the profane; day and night; light and darkness. In Judaism, Christianity, and Islam, a Sabbath day is singled out as special in contrast to the secular weekdays. In fact, most religions have holy days distinct from "every days."

Presumably, whether boundaries relate to physical shelter, our minds, our professions, or our spirituality, they help make us feel secure. What are we, therefore, to make of and how are we to handle ourselves in the face of boundaries that are more amorphous, such as those that come with homelessness or mental illness? Structures we may take for granted may not be accessible to certain individuals, at certain times of their lives. Not fully comprehending the shifting grounds characterizing others' daily lives may trigger some feelings of insecurity of our own.

There's a teaching cited in both the Hebrew Bible (Deut 10:16, 30:6) and the New Testament (Rom 2:29) that may provide some helpful guidance for us here. It instructs listeners to cut away the figurative barrier that shuts out the tenderness of our hearts. When we encounter people and situations whose lives and circumstances challenge our own norms, perhaps what we need to do is to examine whether there are boundaries we set up that are too *im*permeable, too hard to penetrate. While we need to be attentive to maintaining appropriate professional boundaries, are there instances in which we internally set up blockades that are too rigid? In our work with home care patients, we will be challenged by people and circumstances that puncture values we take for granted. Even as the human tendency may be to erect barriers against the things that make us feel insecure or uncomfortable, our challenge is not to lose sight of ways we can soften our hearts. Perhaps we are called not only to maintain professional boundaries, but also to cultivate boundless compassion.

Contemplations

- How would I characterize healthy boundaries in contrast to hard-heartedness?
- What relational barriers do I erect when I feel insecure or uncomfortable?
- Are there ways I can/should soften my heart?

An Affirmation for Me

As one who cares for those who suffer, I am called to maintain professional boundaries as well as to cultivate boundless compassion.

A Prayer to Share

Create in me a pure heart, God, and renew a steadfast spirit within me. Ps 51:10

> God,
> Source of my protection,
> The veil has worn thin
> Between my strength and vulnerability,
> Safety and danger,
> Calm and fear.
> Thoughts and feelings fill me and spill over.
> The unknown feels ominous,
> Unfurling mysteriously into the future,
> And at the same time,
> Gnawing within me.
>
> Please protect me now.
> Even as my body and being are weary,
> My call to You is pure.

Part 1: Vignettes

Renew a steadfast spirit within me.
As I entrust bones and soul
To Your tender care,
Gird me, join me, assure me.
You temper danger and fear—
I may be exposed,
But with You, I am safe.
Your boundless compassion
Puts my heart at ease.

ANDI: CHANGEOVER

Grasping at, insisting on, and analyzing the clear logic of why and how a loved one needs to change does not necessarily make it so, and probably does not *usually* make it so. At least that has been my personal experience as well as my observation of family dynamics in the majority of households I visit. One family member wants so badly for another to behave differently, that this becomes their fixation. Recent back-to-back visits with one of my patients, Andi, perfectly illustrate how this issue can be at the heart of these individuals' spiritual distress.

Andi is a sixty-one-year-old divorced mother of two grown daughters. She was hospitalized recently for an infection related to infusions she receives twice a week for a chronic health condition. These draining medical treatments leave Andi with little energy for much else. She used to be a very active woman—swimming and running daily, working full time since completing college and graduate school, and raising her daughters, for the most part, as a single mother. Today, she lives alone in a single room, undecorated, and minimally furnished apartment that is difficult for her to keep up.

In my first visit with Andi, it wasn't the physical challenges that were sapping her energy and well-being, but her incessant mental reliving of tense episodes and exchanges with her younger daughter, twenty-eight-year-old Ellen. Andi would review hurtful complaints Ellen made toward her as a teenager, dwell on Ellen's lack of responsiveness to her in recent months, and recount the many slights and disappointments in the years in between.

I was surprised during my second visit with Andi that she mentioned nothing about Ellen. Instead, distress immediately poured from her with regard to her older daughter, thirty-two-year-old Jenny. Two days after my initial visit with Andi, Jenny had given birth to her sixth child, by a sixth father. Jenny's story, and Andi's anger and frustration with her, became the central focus of our second conversation.

It was hard to get words in during either of my visits with Andi as her stories and feelings surged forcefully from her. What was clear was that, while anything is possible, it was unlikely that Andi's repeated admonishments of her daughters would change their behaviors to her satisfaction.

In considering counseling around change, I'm reminded of how my thinking progressed over my many years as a hospice chaplain. At first I framed my role as one who assists others in their grief, then I expanded my orientation to see my role as assisting others in their losses. It's not just anticipating death or mourning a loved one that can create emotional and spiritual suffering, but all the losses that often emerge for those nearing end of life, such as loss of independence, mobility, or mental clarity. As time went on, I realized that what I most needed to help others with is change. For example, a grandfather I knew experienced loss around his role as patriarch of his family as he became increasingly frail and dependent on others. His situation was not all about loss, however. With "change" as the touchstone for processing his situation, additional perspectives emerged. Difficult situations often reflect qualities of both shadow and light. For this grandfather, the light emerged by his learning to embrace the gift of receiving, of being cared for by loved ones.

For Andi, like many home care patients, change is front and center. Even when patients have many years ahead of them, the struggles that landed them in home care may reflect conditions that will challenge them to adjust their lifestyles in fundamental ways. Certain realities will be beyond their control, and the only thing they will be able to change will be their own attitudes and priorities. With my encouragement, as Andi processed the dynamics with her daughters, it became increasingly clear to her that she needed to focus more on what nurtures her own emotional well-being and how to make pursuit of inner peace a priority in her life. We did not dismiss her grief and feelings of loss. They are very real and present. Experiences, like this one with Andi, tell me that when we invite those for whom we care to name the changes that really will make a difference to their well-being, we become agents and advocates for a kind of healing that can penetrate body and soul.

Contemplations

- When have I welcomed change in my life? When have I not done so?
- What feelings do I associate with change?
- What is the hardest thing about change?
- How can I best support those I care for through change?

An Affirmation for Me

When confronted with change, though I may not be able to alter specific facts and circumstances, I still can respond in ways that are life-nurturing and healing.

Navigating Changes, Boundaries, and Borderlines

A Prayer to Share

To everything there is a season, a time for every purpose under the sun. Eccl 3:1

> There is a sameness and a newness to each day,
> But change is inevitable—
> Changes that are hard, and changes that are easy;
> Changes I welcome, and changes I resent;
> Changes that bring growth, and changes that leave me feeling stuck;
> Changes I understand, and changes that mystify me;
> Changes I believe others should make, and changes I want to make in myself;
> Changes I embrace, and changes I don't want to speak about;
> Changes that are instantaneous, and changes that happen over time;
> Changes that comfort, and changes that disturb;
> Changes I feel I can control, and changes I know I cannot;
> Changes that inspire, and changes that depress;
> Changes that leave me conflicted, and changes that challenge me to make peace.

CASEY, JACK, RENA, AND DOT: FALLING

When I visited fifty-four-year-old Jack, recently returned home after hospitalization for a pelvic fracture, I immediately noticed his red socks as he stood to greet me. In the hospital, red socks are worn by patients at risk for falling. Now at home, Jack continued to enjoy these bright socks. However, as he wobbled and wavered on his feet, I could see that the red alert should still be active.

Jack was the fourth patient I saw within two days for whom falling is a central concern. First there was Casey who is recovering from a stroke. She is dealing with stressful conflict with her daughter who doesn't like to be woken up at night to assist her mother to the bathroom. Without assistance, however, Casey is in danger of falling. Next was Rena. Although she expects to walk again, currently she is in a wheelchair following injuries due to a fall several months ago. Third was Dot. Dot typically falls once or twice a week. She can't bend her knees properly, so she can't get up on her own. Because she lives alone, she calls 911 whenever she falls. The local firemen come and help her back up.

It's not just our patients who fall. My student, on crutches for a leg injury, recently slipped on some drops of water and fell, potentially making her recovery more protracted. A few years ago, for no identifiable physical reason, at the bedside of a patient I was visiting at the VA Hospital, I mysteriously drifted from standing upright to being collapsed on the floor. I went to college in a small Ohio town. On the coldest, iciest days, you couldn't walk through campus without witnessing a few students taking a spill on the treacherously icy sidewalks. Unlike what we encounter with our patients, the scene of students in their teens and twenties slipping and falling across the quad had the flavor of a slapstick comedy rather than ominous foreshadows of a health decline. Babies, learning how to walk, fall all the time. We expect this and accept it as a normal part of human development.

Perhaps because of our vulnerability to falling, we "normalize" the experience by co-opting the word for scores of metaphors. For instance, we *fall* in love or *fall* head over heels; *fall* from grace; start to cry and *fall* apart; have *a falling* out with someone to whom we used to be close; see a companion's face *fall* after being humiliated; *fall* off the wagon; *fall* into temptation; *fall* asleep. We even imbue a quarter of our calendar year with the nuances of falling by calling the season itself *Fall*. There are dozens of verses in the Bible in which characters "*fall* on their faces"—whether in worshipful prostration or as a shocked reaction to their comrades' behavior.

Effectively, the fact that we all fall, and fall in all kinds of ways, is commonplace. Less universal are the ways we get up. The question becomes, "Once we fall, how will we wake up?" How do we renew ourselves, reestablish a relationship, adjust to new physical challenges, pull ourselves together, or recommit to living up to our highest potential?"

There's a Japanese proverb that says, "Fall down seven times, stand up eight." In our work as home care clinicians, we assist patients in relearning to stand, to walk again, or to get up and become mobile in other ways. We know how falling typically affects patients on many other levels, as well. They may suffer from feelings of lowered confidence or diminished sense of purpose. They may need to adjust to new dependencies on caregivers. Even as we help our patients maneuver with walkers or wheelchairs or assess the adequacy of pain medications prescribed for bruises and broken bones, we also can be companions to them in their struggles to discover how to pick themselves up and re-embrace the potential for meaningful living.

Contemplations

- What is a memorable experience of falling that has happened to me?
- What thoughts and emotions do I associate with that experience?
- What have I learned about "getting back up?"
- What are ways I can best support those for whom I care when they fall?

An Affirmation for Me

I remind myself of the importance of going slowly and gently when recovering from a fall. It takes time to rebuild a trusting relationship with the body or to renew sturdiness of the spirit.

Part 1: Vignettes

A Prayer to Share

You support all who fall, and lift up all the downtrodden. Ps 145:14

> I can't quite fathom how it is, why it is,
> that I find myself on the ground.
> The fall happened so quickly, unexpectedly.
> I was caught off-guard.
> Between feeling sure of myself, and then,
> feeling broken and damaged,
> Something happened.
> I feel out of control. Betrayed. Scared.
> How can I trust myself—to live confidently in mind, body, and spirit?
> I didn't choose to fall;
> it happened without my assent.
> You, God, are the One who supports the falling,
> You are the One who lifts up the downtrodden.
> You raise me up when I falter,
> and sustain me when I am bent over and burdened.
> I can choose to let go now, to release myself into Your embrace.
> You are there to meet me, to catch me.
> Be not only my companion through these low moments,
> But also be my guide.
> With Your help, I trust that I can get up again.

ELSA: WHAT HAPPENS NEXT?

During my first visit with Elsa, she openly shared with me the harrowing details of her early life. A Holocaust survivor, she described her escape from what had seemed sure death. I listened as she described how toward the end of the war on a death march out of Auschwitz, she dove into some bushes on the side of the road. Only she and two other escapees from the march survived. She went on to tell me that she was the only one of 1,500 Jews from her small German town to make it back alive.

On my second visit, our conversation turned to what happens next, after we die. Now one hundred years old and dealing with multiple health issues, Elsa knows that her life is winding down, that she will not live much longer. She pointed to the ground, indicating that that's where we go. "And that's it," she commented. "I'm realistic," she added in her still detectable German accent.

In reflecting on my visits with Elsa, the twentieth-century painter Jackson Pollack comes to mind. Pollack was well-known for his unique artistry technique—splatters of paint across a canvas, conveying randomness and intentionality at the same time, chaos and order—an effect that can be both beautiful *and* unsettling. For the healthcare provider, holding a patient's conflicting palette of ideas in harmonious tension can be its own beautiful *and* unsettling challenge.

With her initial reflection on "what happens next," Elsa painted a first theme on our conversational "canvas"—that there is nothing after we die. Our exploration continued with a discussion about how some people believe they will be reunited with loved ones after death. "That would be nice," Elsa sighed. "I'd like to see my parents again."

"If you were to see them again, what would you say?" I asked. She responded without missing a beat, "Why did you leave me here? Why didn't you take me with you?" After a pause, she reflected, "I don't know why I'm still here." Another pause. "But . . . you go with God when God is ready for you."

With these comments Elsa painted a second theme—that after we die, we do live on, at some level. I responded, "What's interesting to me is that you say there's nothing after we die, but you also say that we go with God. If there's nothing else, then who "goes with God?"

She smiled faintly at my question, catching the tension in the themes she was painting. Eventually, she circled back to where we began. "No," she replied, "to say there's something after we die, that's a fairy tale."

Toward the end of our visit, Elsa again mentioned how "God takes you when God is ready." Back and forth she went—after we die, there is nothing, and after we die, we go with God. Across her emotional and spiritual canvas, Elsa painted a complexity of musings, questions, confusions, assumptions, contradictions, hopes, and disappointments. Her intermittent smiles and the hug she gave me at the end of our visit suggested that being invited to illustrate with all her "colors" was a relief.

In reflecting back on my visit with Elsa, I visualized poignant details of our interaction. To sit with a patient through an impassioned though artful process of self-expression can be unsettling, but also astonishingly beautiful.

Contemplations

- What does the canvas of my spiritual life look like?
- What colors, shapes, images, and words do I include? (Better yet, go ahead and paint it!)

An Affirmation for Me

In accepting that chaos and order live in tension with each other, I will navigate the world with more equanimity and will appreciate its divine complexity.

A Prayer to Share

At the beginning of God's creating of the heavens and the earth—the earth being unformed and void, with darkness over the surface of the deep and the spirit-wind of God sweeping over the water—God said, "Let there be light"; and there was light. Gen 1:1–3

>   Merciful God,
>   Distant Decree-er,

Navigating Changes, Boundaries, and Borderlines

Divine Friend,
Exquisite Challenger—
You create, ordain, grant, and sustain;
Visible and invisible,
Revealing and concealing,
You gift us with freedom and trust.
Source of darkness and wind,
Water and light,
Please notice me and tend to me—
My darkness is enveloped
Within Your darkness.
Form me, re-form me, renew me.
Your light ignites my hope.
There was light,
There is light,
There will be light.
I am very good.

VI.

Standing with Authenticity, Blessed with Revelation

Hospitality is one of the most precious gifts caregivers can bring to those we serve. By this, I mean the willingness to receive and accept others for who they are, to invite their authentic selves to come forth and be seen and appreciated. Being given the time and space to reveal a fuller spectrum of one's achievements, hopes, dreams, disappointments, and regrets can be healing. To be able to reveal oneself to a trusted and caring individual can be a balm. With revelation can come blessing.

TONY: DIGNITY

An oft-repeated lament I hear from patients is how their disease is causing them to lose their dignity. They may no longer be able to do things for themselves the way they used to, they may see themselves as a burden to friends and family, or they may not have control over intimate bodily functions. In this vignette I return to Tony, the forty-two-year old man diagnosed with ALS. He is married to Melinda, and has two sons—ten-year-old Darryl and twelve-year-old Mason.

Standing with Authenticity, Blessed with Revelation

On my third visit with Tony and Melinda, Tony shared this story. After several months of Darryl and Mason not really having a clear picture of their father's illness and his inevitable decline, Tony was home alone with them. He had to use the toilet, but it had come to the point where he was no longer able to dress himself afterward. He would need his sons to assist him. All were uncomfortable. Tony explained how, due to his illness, they would need to pull together as a family, with everyone helping out. Tony felt it was time to share with them the seriousness of the disease. Following his explanation, his younger son Darryl said, "But you're not going to get worse, Dad, right?" Tony explained how he would continue to have less and less control over his body, even as his mind stayed who he has always been. "But," Tony told them, his voice breaking with emotion, "this doesn't mean I love you any less." While he and Darryl were crying, his older son Mason became reflective, saying, "This will help us grow up, and help us become men."

Up until this visit, Tony had remained stoic while sharing the unfolding developments of his illness and their effects on him and the family. Now as he relayed what happened, the tears flowed, just as they had during the actual interaction with his sons. For the first time in the months since his diagnosis, Tony allowed a full expression of emotion—both with his sons, and again in the retelling of the experience to his wife and me.

When I think of key assumptions about living a spiritual life, a common theme across most religious traditions, is the notion that ultimately we are not in control. Some may identify God as the higher power to which we are submissive. More secular-oriented individuals may frame things a bit differently—for example, focusing more on how humans are subject to the forces of nature. Whatever our beliefs, a spiritual life—if characterized as embodying peace and centeredness—typically includes some notion of the need for humble surrender to and acceptance of those circumstances that are beyond our control. I'm not talking about complacence in the face of injustices or apathy in the wake of challenge. I refer to coming to peace with the inevitable, and beyond that, to being attentive to moments of grace and gratitude amidst challenge and suffering.

Tony indeed has lost control over so many of life experiences that he once took for granted. Does that mean he has lost his dignity? If dignity means no need for help with personal bodily care, then yes, he has lost his dignity. If we accept this opinion, then we have undermined essential spiritual values. From a spiritual perspective, dignity isn't something that circumstances can grant or take away. Rather, it is our birthright—inherent to the soul of our humanity—with us until the day we die. It doesn't diminish if our bodies, or even our minds, become broken. In being human, we have dignity. Moreover, love reminds us to trust that this core of our humanity can remain strong until death. Even as his body declines, Tony's dignity soars when he says with a full heart to Daryl and Mason, "This doesn't mean I love you any less."

Contemplations

- How do I understand dignity?
- What enhances dignity? What detracts from it?
- Can a person lose his/her dignity?
- As a clinician/caregiver, how can I support another's feeling of dignity?

An Affirmation for Me

While someone may treat me in an undignified way, or I may find myself in undignified circumstances, no one or no thing can take my dignity away. For in being human, I have dignity.

A Prayer to Share

Set me as a seal upon your heart, as a seal upon your arm, for love is strong as death . . . Song 8:6

> God, I am not who I used to be.
> I used to be whole, strong, capable.
> My life feels diminished now
> by all the things I can no longer do,
> for myself and for others.
> I used to be independent, proudly so.
> And now, I depend on others to assist me, care for me, diagnose me.
> Where is my dignity?
> It feels as if it is slipping through my fingers,
> sliding off my body and being.
> You, God, Who grants dignity, Who is the Giver of life itself,
> Guide me to remember that in bestowing life,
> You bestow dignity.
> You remain true to the gifts You grant.
> No one and no thing can take my dignity, Your dignity away.
> My soul is bound up with You.
> You have created and sustained me with love.
> With You, love remains strong.
> And I remain dignified.
> Love is strong as death.

ANDREW: THE THINGS WE DO FOR LOVE

Do you remember when twenty-six-year-old model Anna Nicole Smith married the eighty-nine-year-old tycoon J. Howard Marshall? The gossip industry speculated she was after his wealth, which she always denied. Marshall died thirteen months later at age ninety, and a battle over his estate ensued.

Part 1: Vignettes

I thought about the Smith–Marshall drama in reflecting on a visit I had with seventy-nine-year-old Andrew. He is a widower with no children or any other family and has chronic health issues that send him in and out of the hospital. Andrew, a retired public service employee, shared the following story with me. A few years ago, he hired a consultant to help him straighten out financial difficulties related to his pension. Diane, the woman he hired, ended up exacerbating the confusion, and he had to hire someone else. However, in the time Diane worked with him, they became friends. In fact, she had been to his home the evening before. She had broken a crystal vase at her own home, wanted one for a party she was having, and knew Andrew would have an extra he could give her. She often admired the many small treasures in Andrew's home, most of which his deceased wife had collected. He felt he didn't need all these possessions and was happy to give things away to someone who would appreciate them.

Recently Andrew revisited his will, making the decision to have Diane inherit the bulk of his estate. After all, he had no family, and she was one of his few friends. He appreciated her coming around to visit and spend time with him. He forgave her for mishandling the pension mess and was glad to have her in his life.

Following my visit, a song went through my mind—"The Things We Do For Love." It's not exactly a sacred hymn in the traditional sense, but the lyrics captured a synthesis of my experience listening to Andrew's story.[1] When we feel lonely or brokenhearted, there may be a lot we will do for love . . .

Andrew is alert and oriented, clear-minded and intelligent. I don't assess that he is a victim of financial abuse. With Diane, he is making a choice. The obvious judgment is that this man is being manipulated. Is he really? In Andrew's relationship with Diane, he *feels* loved.

Sometimes I need to remind myself that people are free to make their own choices, and that it is not my role to judge. I cannot truly understand how others experience love and what they are willing to do for it.

1. Gouldman and Stewart, "The Things We Do for Love."

What I can recommit to is authenticity in my own way of being. Being present with patients with as much authenticity as I can gives them the experience of being *genuinely* cared for. They can have at least one relationship in their lives in which someone isn't *needing* them to be a certain way. Finally, I can be inspired by my work to look at my own intimate relationships. How pure is my own love?

Contemplations

- In caregiving relationships, how have my own choices differed from those for whom I've cared?
- How do I assess when a compromise in a relationship is justified?
- Have I made compromises I later regretted?
- On a scale of 1 to 10—with 1 being "nonjudgmental" and 10 being "most judgmental"—where do I see myself and why?
- Am I content with where I have placed myself on the judgmental scale? Explain.

An Affirmation for Me

In being present with patients as *authentically* as I can, I offer the experience of being *genuinely* cared for.

A Prayer to Share

My sacrifice to God is a broken spirit; God, you will not despise a broken and contrite heart. Ps 51:17

> With the challenges I face now,
> I feel lost and bewildered—

How am I to serve You, God;
How am I to live according to Your will?

People the world over make sacrifices each day,
Whether relational, financial, health related,
In dedicating time and effort to reach a goal,
Or in service to a higher purpose.
I have made sacrifices, too.

But now all I have to offer You, God,
Is my broken spirit and my broken heart.
This is my sacrifice today.
I am blessed in Your assurance
That nothing is more precious to You
Than when Your creatures
Come before You with all who they are,
However that might be.
I am created in Your image,
My Divine, Wounded Creator—
With Your gift of grace,
I am exactly who You need me to be.
You love me for who I am;
And accept what I have to offer today.

BERT: DESERT MINDFULNESS

How do you cultivate that expression of spirituality associated with mindfulness and introspective self-awareness when mental focus feels impossible? Such was the conundrum of Bert, a sixty-seven-year-old man, on Home Care for complications related to an auto-immune disease. Between pain, fatigue, and medications, Bert finds he is unable to concentrate enough to engage in the meditation practice to which he had been committed for the past twenty-plus years. Over the decades, he also has taken great inspiration from esoteric spiritual literature. He would read and contemplate the writings and then assess how best to integrate the teachings into his own life. Lately, even skimming the newspaper is a challenge, let alone engaging the complexities of sacred and philosophical texts.

Alongside a rich history of spiritual practice, Bert had been an accomplished businessman—an inventor and entrepreneur. His successes contributed to a level of financial prosperity that allowed him to own a beautiful, well-appointed home with an ocean view. Similarly to the slipping away of his spiritual practice, his material wealth is unraveling. He has made poor business decisions in the last few years, is not inventing anything new, and expenses related to his deteriorating health are draining his savings. Having divorced six years ago, Bert would like to pursue a new romantic relationship, but doesn't believe he would be attractive to women in his current condition. Spiritually, vocationally, financially, and relationally, Bert feels adrift. He wonders what meaning and purpose his life could have now.

While for Bert the word "adrift" can have negative connotations, a related word, "non-attached," can have positive ones. Buddhism especially lifts up "non-attachment" as a key spiritual pursuit, and considers attachment to be the root of all suffering. In the Hebrew Bible, a non-attachment-like experience also is highlighted as being spiritually pivotal. The Israelites' forty years of wandering in the desert established the groundwork for their readiness to enter the Promised Land.

In many ways, Bert is circumnavigating a kind of desert. He is not able to rely on signposts that have guided him in the past. He has had to relinquish strivings for material success and professional accomplishments. He has modified his aspirations for establishing a romantic attachment. Spiritually, too, Bert realizes that one can become attached to accomplishment in a way that defeats rather than uplifts. When he views certain spiritual practices and pursuits with rigid notions of what he must attain, he undermines opportunities for insights that may come through the desert sojourn. He may no longer have the concentration to sit and practice meditation for thirty minutes a day, but can he be open to the wilderness of unknowing?

In the Hebrew Bible, Revelation comes during a time of wandering and uncertainty. This sets the stage for eventual passage into the Promised Land. In Buddhism non-attachment is a step along the way to experiencing *Bodhi* or enlightenment. According to Islamic tradition, with death comes the opportunity for the veil to be lifted, for our sight to be made keen (Qur'an 50:22). Maybe dying itself offers the possibility for a higher awareness to emerge. Life may have times of disorientation, but ultimately clarity will prevail. From Christianity's New Testament comes the teaching that "the Spirit comes to the aid of our weakness; for we do not know how to pray as we ought, but the Spirit itself intercedes with inexpressible groanings" (Rom 8:26). This teaching complements the gleanings from the other traditions. Perhaps Bert, though in a compromised state of being, can trust Spirit to come to his aid. Though he may experience life now as permeated with barrenness, might there be a coherent force in the Universe to which he can surrender?

Bert and I concluded our visit with a few minutes of sitting and breathing together quietly. We could call it meditation or call it wandering together through the desert. Either way, we surrendered to whatever might be revealed, and so refortified ourselves with a few moments of purpose and meaning.

Contemplations

- To whom and to what am I attached?
- Are there attachments I have that interfere with my caregiving? If so, how might I loosen my hold on these?
- What deserts have I navigated?
- What have I learned from wandering?
- What best equips me to be at peace with not knowing?

Standing with Authenticity, Blessed with Revelation

An Affirmation for Me

When I sit with others in their unknowing and my own, I offer quiet support, patience, and reassurance, trusting that wandering can lead to new insight.

A Prayer to Share

The Eternal your God has blessed you in all the work of your hands, and known your travels in this great wilderness! These forty years the Eternal your God has been with you, and you have not lacked anything. Deut 2:7

> I understand the gift of life to be a blessing, God.
> But today, blessing seems far away.
> I feel lost, as if wandering through a desert.
> I look for signposts, but none emerge.
> Please help me remember that though I cannot see You,
> that You are there,
> for me, with me.
> While I may not have concrete answers to my questions, my concerns, my worries,
> You still are my guide.
> You signal me today to seek the courage to wander,
> to meet the unknown with trust and faith.
> I am not alone.
> As vast as this wilderness of unknowing is,
> Your boundless spirit fills it.
> Help me to welcome the light of this landscape before me,
> to bask in the vastness of Your love.
> There is no true emptiness
> for You are with me.
> I may be wandering, but I am not alone.
> You are my guide, my love, my insight.

Part 1: Vignettes

HERNANDO, LIZ, AND DORIS: REVELATIONS

When talking about spiritual matters, the word "Revelation" carries significant heft. Many religions teach and discuss the concept of Revelation in different ways. We, in the home care world, may have different ideas about revelation through our day-to-day encounters with patients and families. During a week of visits, these revelations unveiled themselves in my encounters:

- A patient's fifty-four-year-old husband revealed that his incapacitated and seemingly soft-spoken, sensitive wife had been so emotionally abusive prior to becoming ill that he was about to leave her. Now he is her 24/7 caregiver.
- A woman in her forties, awaiting a radical and disfiguring surgery for an aggressively progressing cancer, tearfully pondered how much to share about her condition with her fourteen-year-old daughter who already exhibits signs of emotional stress and psychological instability.
- An eighty-year-old woman with end-stage renal failure and multiple additional health challenges revealed that she had hit such a point of desperation over the weekend that she swallowed the rest of her supply of pain pills. Her intention was to end her life.

Obviously our patients' revelations will impact our interventions and plans of care. To supplement this clinical planning process, I offer the following reflections.

When an *unknown* between two people becomes *known,* it can seem as if everything changes *and* nothing changes—both at the same time. The sun may rise and set, same as it always has, but on a heart, mind, and spirit level, we may be forever changed. When we reveal ourselves in relationship, our way of understanding each other may never be the same. For instance, after a patient reveals a vulnerable truth about himself, a nurse might draw blood as he has on countless prior visits. However, how the nurse and the patient feel about each other may have new depth and poignancy. Similarly, after an inspiring spiritual experience or insight, we may view an everyday occurrence—such as the opening of a flower bud—with renewed awe.

When the unknown becomes known, a new connection is forged. Perhaps that's why those for whom we care share intimate details about what they are going through. They reveal in order to connect, to become less isolated. That's where vulnerability comes into play. Revelations can feel risky. Patients are taking the chance that we will be open to connecting. Ideally, not only will we listen, we will respond. In honoring the revelations that patients share with us, we stand with them on sacred ground. While celestial revelations can be wondrous, they are rare. How fortunate we are in our work to have the sacred opportunity to share in revelation, here on earth, most every day.

Contemplations

- Of what particular daily "revelation" do I regularly take note?
- What revelation by a patient saddened me, and how did I respond?
- What revelation by a patient inspired me, and what did I do with that sense of inspiration?

An Affirmation for Me

In welcoming others to share their hidden truths, I discover how blessed I am to have the sacred opportunity to experience the amazement of revelation, here on earth, most every day.

Part 1: Vignettes

A Prayer to Share

Look, I am doing something new! Now it springs forth; do you understand? I am making a path through the wilderness and streams through the wasteland. Isa 43:19

>Dear God,
>I reveal myself to You,
>Trusting that You safeguard all my secrets,
>And all my sorrows,
>And honor them as sacred.
>You know me, and have known me
>From the moment You breathed life
>Into my soul.
>This is a great comfort.
>
>Every day reveals new things—
>Difficulties and possibilities.
>I am making my way
>Because You journey with me.
>We are traveling this wilderness
>Of life and love,
>Of despair and confusion,
>Of hope and worry,
>Together.
>Thank You for this day,
>For all it has revealed and
>All it will reveal.
>Thank You for being the One
>Before whom I can reveal myself
>Fully and completely.

VII.

Witnessing Growth and Discovery

THOSE WHO OBSERVE CAREGIVERS' efforts may note the many gifts they provide to the patients they serve. However, caregivers typically also will suggest that the work they do has many rewards as well. Chief among these is witnessing others' growth and discovery. "Recovery" may be the official care plan underlying many healthcare interventions. Yet, when individuals cope with a serious illness or injury, even if they become physically healthy again, they never will be quite the same as before the incident came about.

To heal physically can be hard work, requiring great endurance, patience, and persistence. When as caregivers we see that our interactions with patients help them to heal not just in body, but support them in growing emotionally, spiritually, and relationally, we may be filled with gratification and gratitude. What an honor, privilege, and inspiration it can be to journey with individuals who are suffering and then witness them growing and discovering new parts of themselves that expand their world, their wisdom, and their hope—even if their physical illnesses prove intractable or fatal.

Part 1: Vignettes

GARY: TO BE A BLESSING

Gary is a man in his early thirties with an eighteen month-old baby. He has been quite sick off and on—mostly on—for the last two years, with repeated hospital stays. The cause of his illness has mystified doctors, but the symptoms have made themselves all too clear: seizures, shingles, repeated episodes of meningitis, and debilitating nausea. Gary's wife works full time as a nurse and understandably has been getting worn down. The other day she lamented to Gary that she feels as if she has to be both mother and father to their young daughter. Between his mysterious illness and his compromised ability to engage with his family, Gary often experiences waves of grief that seem, at times, about to engulf him.

During a difficult stretch between hospital stays, he and his wife had a quiet moment together. Gary was aware and deeply pained by his wife's suffering as a result of his health challenges, but knew that didn't change a fundamental truth. He said to her, "I'm still your husband. I'm here for you. And you can tell me anything."

What strikes me is that for most of us, even at our most compromised—physically, emotionally, spiritually—we long to matter, we long for our lives and our values to mean something. I'm reminded that in a story embraced by three religions (Judaism, Christianity, and Islam) there is the recognition of the significance of *being a blessing*. The foundational covenant for these three traditions begins with the promise to Abraham that he "will be a blessing" (Gen 12:1–2). While Abraham may have gone forth on one kind of journey, our patients go forth on theirs. By the time we interface with them, they often have left places of comfort and familiarity, finding themselves in new territory—places of uncertainty, and filled with a fear of the unknown. Something we can do for our patients, even in the midst of their turmoil and grief, is to recognize and empathize with the human need for purpose, the need for meaning and for connection. We can honor patients' persistence and determination to continue to be a blessing.

Contemplations

- What blessings do I experience in my life?
- In what ways am I a blessing?
- What words of blessing could I offer to someone for whom I am caring now?

An Affirmation for Me

I pause to notice and appreciate how I am a blessing, and how all around me, blessings abound.

A Prayer to Share

I will make you into a great nation, and I will bless you; I will make your name great, and you will be a blessing. Gen 12:2

> Repertoires of prescriptions define my days:
> Intake and output; rest and activity;
> Effort and patience; engagement and silence;
> Today I advocate for the unconventional,
> And tomorrow trust the experts.
>
> But dear God,
> What do You prescribe for me?
> When to protest; when to surrender;
> When to petition; and when to thank?
>
> While there is much I need,
> It seems I have little to give.
> So please, God, train me in kindness;
> Teach me Your compassion;
> Tenderize my heart to see love, be love,

Extend love.
Even if my body fails me,
Blessings abound.
Even if my heart aches,
Blessings abound.
Even if my thoughts become muddled,
Blessings abound.

Along this journey to
the destination—
One day—You will reveal to me,
You have promised
Blessing.
By the way I live, even now,
I am blessed.
As long as I can be,
I will be
A blessing.

JASMINA: THE LITTLE THINGS[1]

Jasmina is a seventy-nine-year-old woman who immigrated to the United States from Serbo-Croatia decades ago. For the past four years she has lived in a board and care. When I introduced myself to her on my first visit, she repeated my name, "'Susan'—That's a sad name."

"What do you mean?" I asked.

"In my language, *susan* means sad," she explained.

"Could that be right?" I wondered. My Google searches later were inconclusive. Fortunately, I happen to have an acquaintance, also originally from Serbo-Croatia. Marko confirmed that in his language *susan* does mean sad. "But you must understand," he

---

1. Previously published in *Reflective Practice: Formation and Supervision in Ministry*, Vol 37, May 2017.

added, "words for sorrow in my language are like words for 'snow' in Eskimo languages. We have many words for sorrow."

Sorrow indeed characterized much of what Jasmina shared with me. She is recuperating from a disfiguring surgery that removed a cancerous tumor, has become blind in the last several years, has no family in this country, and is often lonely. She expressed how she has lost her will to live. After we explored these experiences, I asked her, "Is there anything that helps when you're feeling down?"

"Breakfast," she replied.

"Breakfast?" I said, inviting her to say more.

"They make really good breakfasts here," she explained.

"Oh?" I responded.

"Yes, with eggs and toast, coffee and juice," she elaborated.

We moved on to discussing her desire to reconnect with her church, but she is not in a position to make that happen. I offered to read her some prayers, and she readily agreed. After getting started, she slowed me down, repeating every line after me.

"The Lord is my shepherd," I said.

"The Lord is my shepherd," she'd repeat.

"I shall not want," I recited.

"I shall not want," she repeated, and so we continued.

When we finished, she requested that we talk about the prayer, line by line, then say the whole prayer again in the pattern of my saying a line and her repeating it. She sought to memorize the prayer, to integrate it within her, to savor the words now in order to know them well enough to savor them later.

I am moved by Jasmina's strategy for coping with her deep suffering: pay attention, notice, appreciate, savor the little things, contemplate. She inspires me to reflect on my own life. Although I do not suffer the way Jasmina does, I can learn from her about slowing down enough to appreciate life's nuances.

Jasmina does notice and experience many nuances of sorrow. Can I notice and appreciate the many shades of sorrow experienced by the patients I visit? My hope for Jasmina is that life's small pleasures, like breakfast and savoring the lines of an age-old prayer, can be a source of comfort and reassurance. My hope for myself is that *I* remember to savor breakfast, as well as the many little joys and delights scattered throughout my day.

A reflection from Jon Kabat-Zinn, founder of Mindfulness-Based Stress Reduction, is quite fitting here. As he teaches, "The little things? The little moments? They aren't little."

Contemplations

- What circumstances cause me to rush?
- What are some consequences when I rush?
- What effect does "slowing down" have on me—physically, emotionally, spiritually?
- What strategies can I implement now for integrating more slowing down in my life?

An Affirmation for Me

When I allow myself time to slow down, I appreciate more of life's intricacies, nuances, complexities, and delights.

A Prayer to Share

Teach us to number our days, that we may gain a heart of wisdom. Psalms 90:12

> God, each day you grant is precious—each moment a gift;
> Yet, with the struggles I face these days,
> It's hard to see the joys, to appreciate the miracles.
> Not enough time, or energy, or will and optimism
> To stop and savor;
> To rest and reflect;

To revel in Your creation.

God, my loving teacher,
Please guide me to slow down, to pay attention,
To note the little delights scattered throughout my day.
Remind me to be grateful for the blessings I do have.

There always will be more tasks to complete,
Obligations to fulfill,
Expectations to meet.
But those won't change the number of days I have before me.

Time does not suspend itself,
If I miss a teaching You provide me or
an instance of beauty You unfold before me.

Teach me to number my days,
To taste, smell, hear, see, feel;
To be mindful of my body and being suffused with breath.

Challenge me to fully engage life's joys and sorrows—mine and others.
You who offers me opportunity for insight,
Lead me to pause enough
To learn all You graciously reveal to me, and
To grow my heart toward wisdom.

KARLA: FEELING LIKABLE, BEING LIKABLE

As she has done for the last seven years, Karla stays in bed most of every day. Karla, who is sixty-years-old, suffers from chronic ailments that so overwhelm her with pain that moving into the living room to sit, even for a few minutes a day, or getting to the shower with help are about all she can handle. Every few weeks, she pushes herself to get out of the house for something special. She did so on

Part 1: Vignettes

Christmas and a few weeks later to visit her brother's home for a celebration in honor of her nephew's college graduation.

My visits with Karla focus on two dominant issues. One is her tense and conflictual relationships with family members. Karla lives with her husband, son, daughter-in-law, and baby granddaughter. She also has another son and a daughter who live in town. Karla tells me stories of interchanges with her family. One was on the visit to her brother's home. Navigating with her walker up the long driveway had been a challenge, and halfway up she sat down for a few moments. Reportedly her husband, becoming impatient with her slowness, yelled at her. She told me she had retorted angrily, "Why would we get a walker with a seat if I wasn't supposed to be able to sit down now and then?" Another example she shared was when her daughter visited and reprimanded her for going into the living room where the family was gathered without brushing her hair or wearing a robe over her nightgown. Karla snapped back, criticizing her daughter's lack of empathy. She also told me how her son admonishes her to keep away from the baby when she bends down to give her a kiss.

After hearing the fourth or fifth of these kind of stories, the thought dawned on me, "Wow, Karla's family doesn't seem to like her very much." It's difficult for me to understand the full scope of this family's dynamics in a visit or two. I can't really know what has happened over the years and who has contributed what to the alienated feelings among family members. I listen, offer support and empathy to Karla, and reflect with her on ways to improve communication.

The second issue is her anger with God, a topic she moves toward after our discussion about family issues. Karla was raised Catholic, but hasn't felt connected to the Church in many years. However, she thinks about God, engages with God, even as much of that engagement is dismay. "If I accept that God is an all-powerful God, then how could God allow so much suffering?" she challenges. I explore with her other ways of understanding God's role and power that also harmonize with her faith background—for instance, seeing God not as the source of our suffering but as

One who is *with* us in our suffering, as One who hears our prayers and understands our travails. Karla was open to this theological exploration and welcomed my offer to read to her from a booklet of spiritual reflections. I read one called, "God Loves Me," and another called, "Let Go, Let God." She listened intently and wondered out loud why she had forgotten that God loves her. When I visited the next week, Karla pointed out other readings in the booklet that she had found deeply meaningful. They had themes such as leaning on God, forgiving, and being enfolded in God's presence. It seemed Karla was testing the possibility and then beginning to remember that she is lovable.

This idea of being lovable relates back to Karla's family and their dynamics. Again, the complexities will not resolve themselves overnight, but my hunch is that for Karla's family to like her, it would help for her to *see herself* as likable. Consider the famous teaching, "Love your neighbor as yourself" (Lev 19:18). An implication is that you need to love *yourself* as the starting point for loving your neighbor. Presumably to have the resources to love, the resources to like and to be liked, requires you to like yourself. In other words, to *be* likable, you have to *feel* likable. Though never stated explicitly, Karla and I contemplated this insight through our spiritual conversation. For other patients, the approach may be more humanistically rather than theologically focused. Either way, my conclusion is that a worthy plan of care for a patient such as Karla is to create a safe space for inhabiting the experience of feeling likable. To *be* likable, you have to *feel* likable.

Contemplations

- What do people like about me?
- What do I like about myself?
- How does feeling loved or unloved affect my relationships with others?
- What are ways for me to cultivate self-love?

PART 1: VIGNETTES

An Affirmation for Me

Being attentive to self-love means having more love to give others.

A Prayer to Share

I am my beloved's and my beloved is mine . . . Song of Solomon 6:3

> I am loved because You created me.
> I am loved because when I hid from You,
> You called me;
> Assuring that we are bound together
> Within and beyond Eternity's garden.
> I am loved because You see me for all who I am,
> Naked or clothed,
> Exposed or defended—
> It doesn't matter to You.
> I am loved because when floods have come—
> Floods of worries or floods of sorrow;
> Floods of regret or floods of disappointment;
> You are my raft,
> Inviting me aloft when troubles threaten.
> I am loved because—when there is no "because" to grasp,
> No explanation to satisfy—
> You hear me, understand me, know me.
> I am Yours and You are mine.
> With You as my beloved, today and always—
> I am enough.

CECILE: ACCOUNTING FOR VULNERABILITY

Cecile is a sixty-four-year-old woman being treated for wounds incurred after a dog attack. Besides the trauma of the assault by an animal that she had lived with and cared for two years, Cecile feels grief and guilt about her family's decision to euthanize the dog. The seriousness of her wounds makes it difficult for her to get up and move around or to use her hands. The healing process will take several months.

Cecile is not used to sitting around while others serve her and care for her. She is the matriarch of a household that includes three generations. It always has been her role to be caregiver—to clean, shop, cook, and address the many demands of her active family. Along with the distressing circumstances surrounding her injuries, being so limited in how she typically engages in life makes Cecile feel very vulnerable. Given her new experience of spending many hours in quiet and stillness, Cecile feels compelled to explore these vulnerable feelings.

It's hard for her to recognize herself—not just physically and emotionally, but relationally and spiritually. Cecile finds herself questioning unhealthy relational dynamics that up until now she had ignored, as well as not sufficiently appreciating the good in other relationships she took for granted. Cecile wonders how she drifted away from the faith of her youth, the faith that at one time was so meaningful to her. She questions whether she wants to return to her religious roots or explore other spiritual paths. In slowing down, she has come to recognize that over the years she has not allowed herself sufficient space and time to address her own personal emotional issues, to nurture and appreciate some relationships and address problems in others, or to cultivate her own authentic spiritual expression.

Cecile experiences her vulnerability as both uncomfortable *and* motivating. Not everyone responds to such acute feelings of vulnerability with the sense that he or she has a potential opportunity for growth and change. I affirm her courage. A temptation with vulnerability is to run away from it. Another response, Cecile's response, is to do the exact opposite: to go toward it, to take an accounting of all the agitations the vulnerability stirs up. I'm reminded of a valued spiritual process in my tradition called *soul accounting*. Soul accounting requires commitment to penetrating introspection and self-examination. This process can bring profound self-growth, but it's not easy.

I can't imagine anyone welcoming the physical pain and emotional trauma that come with as terrible an experience as Cecile went through. However our lives unfold though, the circumstances dealt us present a "soul accounting" opportunity. By moving *toward* the vulnerability, we open ourselves to insight and wisdom that otherwise may not have been accessible to us. Discomfort can transform into motivation to learn and to grow, and to make life-affirming changes.

For Cecile, her "soul accounting" spans personal emotional issues, relationship concerns, and neglected spirituality. Her accounting has stimulated ideas for facing difficult realities and envisioning effective strategies for addressing them. A challenge for those who visit with individuals like Cecile is to be willing to journey with them to their spaces of vulnerability. Can we be comfortable enough with ourselves to be present with others in their discomfort? One way to cultivate our ability to do so is to commit to making "soul accounting" a part of our own lives; that is, to recognize *our own* vulnerability, go toward and embrace it, and appreciate the gifts it can teach.

Contemplations

- What makes me feel vulnerable?
- How do I deal with my own feelings of vulnerability?
- What are my responses to others' vulnerability?
- How would I design a process of "soul accounting" for myself?

An Affirmation for Me

I am willing to journey to spaces of vulnerability—mine and those of others—to embrace and appreciate the insights that will emerge.

A Prayer to Share

God, when you favored me, you made my royal mountain stand firm; but when you hid your face, I was troubled. Ps 30:7

Turn us to You, God, and we will return . . . Lam 21:5

>God, where did the time go when I felt solid,
>When my body and being could stand tall and firm?
>You may have made me in Your image,
>But if You meant to make me whole and complete,
>I do not feel that way.
>I feel broken and hardly recognize myself.
>Who are You, that I reflect Your Image?
>Do not remain hidden.
>
>I seek Your wholeness and completeness,
>But You respond—
>As long as any of Your creatures are broken,
>You, too are broken.
>As long as I cry, You cry.
>As long as I fear or hurt or despair,
>Your very being reverberates with my emotion.
>
>I thought You hid from me,
>But I hid from You,
>And I was troubled—
>I could no longer see You.
>Guide me to reveal my face to You,
>To reveal my heart, my tears, my brokenness.
>As long as I turn to You, You no longer are hidden.
>When I turn to You,
>You turn to me.

PART 1: VIGNETTES

GARY: WHAT CHOICE DO WE HAVE?

In the first vignette in this section, I told a story of my first visit with Gary, a thirty-three year-old married man with a young child. I shared about how important it was for him to "be a blessing" despite all the limitations he experienced due to his health problems. After many months of debilitating illness, at home and in the hospital, Gary finally had recovered enough to be discharged from home care.

During what was to be my last visit with Gary, he reflected on the past months and what he had learned from being ill. I was touched by his intentionality in identifying the positive effects of the insights he had gained. He had re-evaluated his priorities in major categories of his life—the centrality of quality time with his family; keeping more healthful and manageable boundaries in his work life; reassessing which friendships were nurturing and which were draining; and making his personal spirituality and affiliation with a worship community more integral to his life. For all the trials and trauma of the last months, Gary chose to look at his experience in as optimistic a light as possible, to express gratitude for how he had been changed for the better because of what he had gone through.

As I listened to and supported Gary in his reflecting, I felt inspired by his upbeat and grateful attitude. At the same time, then as now, I can't help but wonder: Why, when faced with trying times, do some people focus on the blessings, the lessons and opportunities for growth and insight; while others tend toward self-pity, anger, resentment, despair, or seeing themselves as victims? One possible answer is that some people are more naturally positive—it's just part of their personalities, how they were born. On the other side, biological factors underlying certain mental health diagnoses may complicate some individuals' ability to control their moods and attitude.

But let's take a person who is not born with a predisposition to optimism and gratitude, nor suffering from clinical depression or other mental illness. To what degree does such an individual have the *choice* to embrace the blessings, to find the meaningful lessons amidst the trials? There's a biblical passage that exhorts listeners to choose what is life-giving, to choose blessing over curse—insinuating that we have the capacity to choose where we direct our energy, what priorities we set, and how we view setbacks (Deut 30:19).

I suggest that if we wait until the crises happen to seek and embrace the blessings amidst the curses and to access the life-giving lessons, we likely will come up short. To face life's most daunting challenges with maximum grace requires cultivating the trait of *choosing blessing* each and every day. We have to practice! Looking for and embracing the good in the *daily* ups and downs means that when a crisis hits, we will have cultivated the resources to open our minds and hearts wider to appreciate the lessons, insights, and wisdom that may be buried beneath the pain.

How does all this translate to patient care? I don't suggest explicitly thrusting our own endeavors for personal growth onto the patients whom we serve. I do believe, however, if we practice choosing life and blessing in our daily experiences, those whom we care for will pick up on our attitude and energy, and perhaps grow in *their* courage to see and experience their own circumstances with more insight and wisdom.

Contemplations

- Where do I place myself on a scale of 1 to 10, with 1 being less naturally inclined toward gratitude, and 10 being most highly inclined?
- What gratitude practices do I have now?
- What gratitude practices would I like to cultivate?
- How does gratitude affect my relationships—both gratitude I extend to others and gratitude others extend to me?

Part 1: Vignettes

An Affirmation for Me

When I *choose blessing* through seeking the good within life's inevitable ups and downs, I grow in appreciation for lessons, insights, and wisdom that may be buried beneath life's painful moments.

A Prayer to Share

I call heaven and earth as witnesses against you this day, that I have set before you life and death, blessing and curse. Now choose life, that you and your children may live. Deut 30:19

> God, my life feels confined—
> My living space; what I do and can't do; what I eat;
> When to rest, and when to get up;
> Who I must listen to; plans of care . . .
> It used to be when work and chores were complete,
> I spent my time as I pleased.
> Now medication timetables, therapies, and appointments
> Fill my hours;
> A prescription of "Do's and Don't's" define my days.
> How do I live with my disappointments and dashed hopes?
>
> You, God who created the good and the very good,
> Help *me* to see the good,
> To seek the good, despite the curses;
> Teach me to name the blessings, hidden amidst the suffering;
> Guide me to embrace the lessons,
> Receive the insights, and warm to the wisdom
> Buried beneath the pain.
> However I may live, and whenever I may die,
> Imbue me with the capacity to bless.
> In choosing life, I bind myself to You,
> Source of Life;
> In choosing blessing, I align myself with You
> Who are the Promise and Peace of Eternal Life.

PART 2

Reflections and Theories

VIII.

Spiritual Pain: Theirs and Ours

Human beings are inter-connected. We are made for relationship. Our interconnectedness means we likely will identify with some of our patients' circumstances. Both scientific research and common human experience reveal how humans "catch" each others' emotions. Most of us have been in situations when one person giggling or yawning seems to provoke parallel responses in others. An extreme version of "laughter contagion" took place in Tanganyika (now Tanzania) in 1962. In this case a laughter epidemic spread from a few girls in a boarding school to over a thousand people. Consider, as another example, the adage that as a parent, you are only as happy as your least happy child. That is, a child's unhappiness likely will create a ripple effect of unhappiness in the child's parents. Surely most people recognize instances in which our own eyes well up with tears when we witness another person suffering.

SOURCES OF SPIRITUAL PAIN

We share in each others' pain. In recent decades, numerous studies by psychologists, neurologists, and social scientists have focused on the experience of "emotional contagion." These studies explore how humans can become emotionally involved with each other.

Part 2: Reflections and Theories

Richard F. Groves and Henriette Klauser hone in on specific categories that underpin spiritual pain.[1] They submit that spiritual pain results from a lack of meaning; a sense of "un-forgiveness" either of self or others; feeling alienated from someone/something important in one's life; or hopelessness. In short, the categories are: 1) meaning, 2) forgiveness; 3) relatedness; and 4) hope. Although the vignettes I have described in this book are not necessarily explicit in naming these concerns, the reader will see these themes popping up throughout the telling of the stories. It is not uncommon for our own spirits to be touched deeply by the pain felt and expressed by those for whom we care.

From a mental health perspective, existential psychotherapists such as Irvin Yalom discuss the human need to address what Yalom called "ultimate concerns": death, freedom, isolation, and meaninglessness.[2] Theorists in this school of thought may or may not label these concerns as sources of spiritual pain. Nevertheless, the resonance is obvious—between existential psychotherapy, and the four experiences of spiritual pain Groves and Klauser identify: meaning, forgiveness, relatedness, and hope. From the existential humanist point of view, psychological and emotional suffering cannot be alleviated if "ultimate concerns" go unaddressed or ignored. A skilled therapist will assist the client in negotiating complex feelings around death, freedom, isolation, and meaninglessness. It is hard to imagine a person living a life of well-being without coming to at least a modicum of peace around these matters.

Protestant theologian Paul Tillich also theorized about and used the term *ultimate concerns*.[3] He identified these as the things that claim ultimacy on us and that condition our very existence. To Tillich, faith and its facets are central. In a faith context, we might include as "ultimate concerns" the larger questions of existence, such as: How do we derive meaning in our lives? How do we make peace with suffering and death? Can we apprehend the mysterious way of the Divine day to day?

1. Groves and Klauser, *The American Book of Living and Dying,* 43.
2. Yalom, *The Gift of Therapy,* xvii.
3. Tillich. *Systematic Theology,* 1:12.

Spiritual Pain: Theirs and Ours

Jewish belief infers meaning as arising from dedication to Torah and *mitzvot*—that is, living by a given set of ethical and spiritual precepts. Alienation from Torah and neglect of *mitzvot* give rise to spiritual pain. For Christians, the life and death of Jesus is the central paradigm for addressing meaning in suffering, and for ascertaining the source of redemption. Faithlessness becomes a key culprit of spiritual pain.

When asked what is the greatest commandment, the New Testament depicts Jesus paraphrasing these Torah teachings: "You shall love the Eternal your God with all your heart, and with all your soul, and with all your might;" and "You shall love your neighbor as yourself" (Deut 6:5, Lev 19:18, Matt 22:36–40). From both Jewish and Christian perspectives, love of God, self, and others are essential to a life of meaning. A major source of spiritual pain is that which arises with deprivation of or estrangement from love. Its healing comes with the nurturing of or the return to loving relationships. The loving-kindness caregivers offer can serve as a conduit for this healing process. For the professional caregiver, the work of loving care is consistent with the most repeated commandments in the Torah. Loving and caring for the stranger is the subject matter no less than thirty-six times!

From the world of Eastern thought, the Yoga Sutras of Pantanjali are just one resource that describes root sources of spiritual pain. Sutra 2:3 outlines these central obstacles *(kleshas)* to the spiritual path, obstacles that provoke suffering:

- *avidya,* ignorance, lack of self-awareness, not seeing clearly;
- *asmita* or entanglement in ego;
- *raga* or attraction attachment;
- *dvesha* or aversion; and
- *abhinivesha* or clinging to life/ fear of death, fear of an ending.

Caregivers, whether they be professionals or family members, likely will come across suffering induced by such obstacles. It may be helpful to explore questions that parallel the *kleshas* such as how might we support others to:

- become more self-aware,
- see themselves and their circumstances more clearly;
- let go of their attachments to expectations;
- overcome self-sabotaging bitterness or antagonism; and
- come to greater peace in accepting the seriousness of a life-threatening health condition?

The more we are alert to potential sources of spiritual pain, the more equipped we will be to respond compassionately when we see such pain emerging in our patients and loved ones as well as ourselves. We will no longer see cries of loneliness, aversion to a particular therapy, ignoring the "facts," distress over a felt sense of purposelessness, and so on as complaints and distractions, but as symptoms of spiritual pain.

Like any other pain, spiritual pain needs to be addressed. Without responding to pain, healing will not take place. To the degree that we all, in the end, are both healers and patients, we would be wise not only to pay attention to spiritual pain but have strategies for addressing it, and most importantly to have compassion for those who show signs of being afflicted by it.

IX.

To Be at Home

Where, when, and how can a home be a conducive environment not only for healing physical ailments, but for working through and overcoming spiritual pain? This section provides some answers to these questions, as well as looks at notions of feeling safe, whole, and at peace; how we might confront and integrate difficult changes and losses; and understandings of the cosmic home or "home-to-come."

FROM BIRTH TO DEATH

In many parts of the world, home is the place where recuperation from illness and rehabilitation from accidents happen. At one time in the United States, this was true as well. Not only was home where one would reside throughout the course of an illness, but it also was the locale for births and deaths. Over the last decades, increasing numbers of families are choosing to return to births at home or at birthing centers designed to be as "homey" as possible. At the other end of the life cycle, as the hospice movement has grown, more and more individuals recognize the value of and express a preference for dying at home.

While families expecting babies have embraced hominess as the ideal environment for births and advocates for dying at home have increased in recent years, hospitals and other professional medical institutions have remained the focal point for convalescence. The gap in approaches appears to be narrowing, however. If we have a serious illness, we still may go to the hospital, but getting out of the hospital promptly and not returning anytime soon is increasingly the ideal. Clearly, there are financial motives for discharging hospital patients as soon as possible and working to prevent relapses that lead to readmissions. Even so, attending to patients at home has a non-financially motivated benefit, as well. For many individuals, being at home can provide the most therapeutic environment and maximize conditions especially conducive to healing.

Whatever the motivation, limiting hospital stays means increasing numbers of often extremely fragile and vulnerable patients will be at home. When newly discharged patients are in such conditions, more intensive and conceivably intrusive levels of assistance within the confines of their once private, personal environment may be necessary. Even using the term *patients* is odd. When people are at home, we typically presume them to be residents. Instead, once they are sick and professionals are called in to help them heal, home residents are renamed patients. For the healthcare clinicians, attending to patients at home has its challenges, which grow with the severity of patients' ailments. Opportunities exist in these challenges as well. Just as our culture is returning to home/hominess as the ideal setting for births and deaths, so too can we embrace the potential blessings for recuperation at home.

HEALING AT HOME

To heal at home requires multifaceted efforts. Healing may require wound management, medication review, infusion procedures, physical therapy, occupational therapy, speech therapy, assistance with bodily care, and/or other interventions. But for individuals to feel healed—to feel safe, whole, and at peace—may require many additional levels of consideration. While after a few weeks of skilled therapy a person may be rehabilitated enough to manage physically at home, loneliness, anxiety, fear, and depression may undermine that person's confidence in the stability of recovery.

Whether one embraces a theologically based faith or has a more humanistic philosophy, the values of being safe, whole, and at peace are seemingly universal. A verse from Psalms says:

> Happy are those who dwell in Your house, continually offering You praise. (Ps 84:5)

I imagine the Psalmist addressing this sentiment to God and envisioning this spiritually paradigmatic house as a refuge in which one feels safe, whole, and at peace. Such an experience would echo what recuperating patients typically need to sustain their sense of embodying healing. The Psalmist's aspiration to "dwell in Your house" is akin to what is presumably a predominant human desire across diverse cultures and faiths—that is, continually to reside in a healing space, both literally and figuratively. When we feel safe, whole, and at peace, our hearts and souls can settle enough to express a litany of praise. The more our society helps ailing individuals cultivate this ideal sense of home, the more sustainable their experience of healing will be. Healthcare clinicians and other caregivers stand at the forefront of this "society."

From another tradition, that of yogic philosophy, come these words that offer a different kind of teaching about home: "When disturbed by negative thoughts, opposite [positive] ones should be cultivated. This is *pratipaksha bhavana*."[1]

One way to translate the Sanskrit words *pratipaksha bhavana* is, "Moving to the other side of the home." *Prati* means "other, opposing;" *paksha* means "wing, half;" and *bhavana* means "dwelling, home, mansion, being." In essence, the sutra counsels that when negativity surges, we must make a change—get ourselves out of one place and go to another. Metaphorically, the implication is that the mind has the capacity to shift its focus from the negative to the

---

1. Pantanjali, "The Online Study Resource for the Yoga Sutras of Pantanjali," Sutra 2:33.

positive. When we re-situate ourselves emotionally and spiritually, we grow in our capacity to reframe entrenched perspectives.

Illness may force modifications in a person's home. For instance, a support bar may need to be added to a bathroom, new diet guidelines may require altering culinary practices, a hospital bed or special mattress may need to be set up. Necessary changes to one's home can arouse mixed feelings. On one hand, there may be negativity: "My home has been depressingly altered to accommodate my disabilities and fragilities." On the other hand, there may be positives: "Due to these changes in my home, I am able to remain here and be safe."

Each stage in illness presents possibilities for getting stuck in the most negative interpretation, for lingering in the "worst room of the house." Likewise, each stage offers opportunities to seek more affirmative accountings of changes, for exploring the "other side of the home." Just as a home may have many wings, or nooks and crannies, the mind has many choices, many "rooms." The yoga sutra teaches that our attitude and thoughts are significant in determining into which room we will settle ourselves. Something healthcare providers and other caregivers can offer is the encouragement to dare to enter new rooms, new spaces.

A well-known passage from the New Testament also refers to the many rooms of a house:

> Let not your hearts be troubled: believe in God, believe also in me. In my Father's house are many rooms. If that were not so, would I have told you that I'm going to prepare a place for you. And when I go to prepare a place for you, I will come again and will take you to be with me; that where I am you may be also. And you know the way where I am going. (John 14:1–4)

For those who have a religious practice, this passage using Christian language touches upon the centrality of faith, and with it the promise of and reassurance in an afterlife. In that next world, that "home-to-come," believers will arrive in a place in which they will fully experience God's loving presence enveloping them. While the yoga sutra is more of a here-and-now instruction, this passage from the New Testament speaks to hope, promise, and faith. Even as the passage is future-oriented, it addresses how our sense of what's next can impact our present coping. When we have hope, our hearts will be more at ease. "Let your hearts not be troubled," says the first verse. When we envision a better future, we are more apt to surrender to, or at least come to realistic terms with, what we are facing now. Feeling more secure in the home inside of ourselves can help make it so that our physical environment and bodily limitations will have less sway in defining us.

HOME AS HOPE

But a theistic faith, with its promise of eternal life, may not speak to everyone. The idea of a future containing many possibilities, many "rooms," does not depend on belief in a specific deity. Cultivating hope is an effort open to all, regardless of a particular faith tradition, and is a means of nurturing resilience now. For some, cosmic hopes (such as being united with God for eternity) will be the most inspiring and consoling. For others, more tangible hopes will make the difference to their day-to-day quality of life (for example, the specific and concrete hope to attend a grandchild's wedding). For still others, a more abstract hope will resonate, such as the belief in their potential for personal growth as a result of coping with illness or disability (for example, developing certain qualities, such as patience, forgiveness, gratitude, or humility).

As the New Testament passage indicates, there may be many rooms out there, into the future, as part of the promise of a joyous afterlife. There are many rooms as well, however, accessible to us in our homes here and now. While many anticipate God eventually guiding us to the cosmic home, there is plenty of "housework" in the meantime to tend to in our earthly lives. To manage day-to-day illnesses and crises, we will need the human efforts required to guide each other. The experience of caring for each other can become a source of hope. When we respond with skills, attentiveness, and sincerity to those who are ailing, we become effective navigators through the world's travails. We lead each other to

Part 2: Reflections and Theories

those peaceful perches, those quiet rooms in which those among us who are recuperating can rest for awhile and heal.

HOME AS PEACE

As alluded to previously, we often associate the ultimate "going home" with dying. Using "home" imagery for envisioning what comes next can diminish fears, as home typically suggests a place of reassuring familiarity. Poet and essayist Kathleen Norris goes as far as to say, "Peace, that was the other name for home."[2] Ideally, peace is the experience to which we ultimately will transition. To the degree that caregivers and clinicians can support patients in cultivating peace throughout their health struggles, the more metaphorically at home patients will feel when they literally are at home, and the less fear they likely will have as they anticipate what happens next, when life comes to an end. On a related note, when hospital or care facility patients come to the end of their lives, caregivers and clinicians can play an essential role in supporting them to feel at home with themselves, even when they are not at home literally.

If illness overwhelms and life becomes increasingly intolerable, the contours of hope may change. Artist Frida Kahlo expressed a sentiment along these lines in a diary entry toward the end of her life. She wrote, "I hope the exit is joyful and i hope never to return."[3] When improving the conditions for recuperating at home becomes more and more difficult and patients begin to turn to relief from suffering as their predominant wish, the role of professional home care providers may need to change. It may no longer be in the patient's best interest for us to continue as temporary, part-time dwellers within that individual's home. We may need to transfer our involvement in our patients' lives to others. Calling upon hospice or other palliative care specialists may become the most supportive intervention. They then will take the

2. Norris, "Spirituality & Health."
3. Last words in Frida Kahlo's diary, July 1954.

lead in accompanying and guiding the dying to the home that is eternal peace.

WHEN THE PHYSICAL HOME IS NOT A PLACE OF PEACE

We just explored facets of home, understood as a physical place, metaphorically—as an inner space—a way of being in the world, and as an ultimate destiny (for some). A challenge is how to think about those for whom a physical home may not be a place of peace, but rather a place of discord, turmoil, or even abuse. For those who live in environments, such as single-residence occupancy housing (SROs), home may feel like a prison of loneliness and isolation. There is much work to be done in our society to ensure an experience of and opportunity for home-as-refuge to those who have limited mental, social, or financial resources. Creative efforts are emerging, but we have a long way to go. If being able to reside in a home that feels safe and peaceful is an integral component of healing, then societal attention to a patient's living environment is an integral requirement of holistic healthcare.

X.

What Can We Do to Serve?

"What Can We Do to Help?" was my original title for this section, but I changed my mind after one of my students brought to my attention a powerful essay by Naomi Rachel Remen. In this essay, "In the Service of Life," Remen suggests that helping incurs debt; whereas serving, like healing is mutual. She says, "I am as served as the person I am serving. When I help, I have a feeling of satisfaction. When I serve I have a feeling of gratitude. These are very different things." Expanding on these thoughts, she adds:

> Our service serves us as well as others. That which uses us strengthens us. Over time, fixing, helping are depleting, draining. Over time we burn out. Service is renewing. When we serve, our work itself will sustain us. Service rests on the basic premise that the nature of life is sacred, that life is a holy mystery which has an unknown purpose. Fundamentally, helping, fixing, and service are ways of seeing life. When you help, you see life as weak, when you fix, you see life as broken. When you serve, you see life as whole. From the perspective of service, we are all connected: All suffering is like my suffering, and all joy is like my joy. The impulse to serve emerges naturally and inevitably from this way of seeing.[1]

---

1. Remen, "In the Service of Life," 2.

Using Remen's wisdom as a framework, what follows are specific considerations and suggestions—qualities, interventions, and skills—for supporting those for whom we care through times of especial vulnerability and/or crisis. To do so may call for us to engage those we serve in identifying touchstones and sources of meaning, peace, hope, forgiveness, courage, connectedness, and reassurance.

QUANTITATIVE SUPPORT—"DOING"

Professional spiritual care providers may draw on specific tools and skills to enhance patient/family coping and well-being. These can include:

- ritual,
- prayer,
- blessing,
- reconciliation,
- counsel,
- life review,
- assistance with reflection on goals/values,
- processing/unraveling an ethical dilemma,
- exploration of ultimate questions and sources of meaning,
- encouragement,
- comforting,
- affirmation of strengths,
- normalization of feelings and experiences,
- making referrals, providing resources,
- identifying role models and inspirational stories/teachings, and
- guidance for integrating psychological dissonance.

Part 2: Reflections and Theories

Non-professionals may not have the formal training in utilizing all these tools. Still, there are several tools that most of those who have provided care to another in need will know about and can develop, tools such as, offering comfort and encouragement, affirming strengths, or extending an invitation to reflect on goals and values.

QUALITATIVE SUPPORT—"BEING"

In their book mentioned earlier, *The American Book of Living and Dying*, Richard Groves and Harriet Klauser define "Ten Commandments for the Anam Cara." *Anam cara* is a soul-friend who serves as a companion to the dying, or more broadly as a trusted spiritual guide. The term comes from Celtic tradition and has a long and rich history. While the preceding paragraph outlines specific activities and interventions for a caring companion to offer, these "commandments" address the more qualitative dimensions for a caregiver to cultivate. Here are Groves and Klauser's suggestions for being a "soul friend":

1. Be present.
2. Trust that who you are is enough.
3. Share with your friends as an equal.
4. Listen rather than being concerned with doing.
5. Pay attention to changing priorities.
6. Pay attention to your needs and feelings.
7. Just keep breathing.
8. Pay attention to the clues.
9. Remember that you are not alone.
10. Grieve and keep remembering.[2]

Suggestions for the anam cara are prescribed particularly for the context of companionship to the dying. Thinking about

2. Groves and Klauser, *The American Book of Living and Dying*, 56–60.

caregiving more broadly, I encourage consideration of another framework. While we may offer support to our patients, ideally, the larger context in which we meet them is as "co-journeyers." The recuperating process perhaps can feel slightly less lonely when a visitor comes and conveys, though not necessarily with words, a message such as this: "I am here to be with you. Let's travel together for a while. Thus, will our spirits be lifted. I will do whatever I can to lift you, but as importantly, you, too, have the power to lift; to lift this moment. You are not alone. As we are present with each other, we share the blessing of transforming an encounter between caregiver and sick person, to an encounter between soul and soul. And in the end, all is soul. You have nothing to fear."

When we, as caregivers attune ourselves to our own spirituality, religious beliefs, and sources of personal meaning, we help equip ourselves to be "co-journeyers." The section "Spiritual Pain" presented a few touchstones that may guide and inspire certain caregivers—for instance, loving your neighbor as yourself, and loving the stranger. Inspiring resources about the value of compassionate and loving care are abundant across religious traditions and humanistic worldviews. We would do well to identify teachings that especially speak to us, teachings that will provide us with guidance, support, affirmation, and reassurance for the challenges and the rewards of caregiving, of serving.

XI.

The Most Potent Intervention

THE PREVIOUS CHAPTER OUTLINED specific interventions—some of which are more reflective of "doing" and others of "being." Woven through many of the interventions is the inference of the importance of attentive listening. To respond effectively to the emotional and spiritual needs of those for whom we care means employing what probably is the most potent intervention—listening.

LISTENING FULLY AND WHOLEHEARTEDLY

Listening fully and wholeheartedly straddles the categories of both doing and being. From our own experiences of being a caregiver or a recipient of care, we have a sense of how powerful listening can be. Many caregivers to whom I talk, whether healthcare professionals, family members, or therapists, tell stories of listening intently to others who are hurting, perhaps saying very little or even nothing during the process. Afterward, these hurting individuals will report feeling much better.

I remember a time when I visited a hospice patient who, upon my inquiry at the beginning of the visit, reported her pain level as a "10." Seeing that she was communicating with me calmly and clearly, I chose to engage with her more before running down the hall for help. We ended up visiting for almost an hour, during which time she shared feelings about her illness, concerns about her family, details about the home she left due to her need to be in a skilled nursing facility, and more. As the visit seemed to be winding down, I returned to the pain question: "What is your pain level now?" I asked. Her response? "Oh, I don't have any pain." I imagine most of us can remember a time in our lives when someone really listened to us. Perhaps we can recall how the gift of being listened to helped alleviate our own pain and suffering—perhaps a little, or perhaps, like the hospice patient I describe, a great deal. Listening can be remarkably healing.

LISTENING TECHNIQUES

Much has been written about listening techniques. An essay by Robert Kidd that I especially appreciate details "foundational listening and responding skills" that a spiritual care provider should master. These include: literal repetition, reflecting, paraphrasing, open-ended questions, buffering, "tell-me-more" and minimal encouragement responses, intense interaction responses, calling attention (highlighting unconscious or seemingly unnoticed reactions or behaviors), and hovering ("over a topic . . . to get a more comprehensive view of the whole").[1]

In their psycho-therapeutic article, "Post-Modern Approaches to Psychotherapy," Robert A. Neimeyer and Sara K. Bridges delineate the following words to articulate strategies for working with clients, most of which explicitly involve close and careful listening: orienting, centering, focusing, empathizing, analogizing, nuancing, dilating, constricting, tacking, contrasting, structuring, ambiguating, weaving, enacting, externalizing, and witnessing.[2]

Resources like those just described provide how-to guidelines for effective listening, detailing actions to take and qualities to cultivate. Other commonly known concrete practices are: maintain good eye contact; sit in a relaxed, open posture; and use

---

1. Kidd, "Foundational Listening and Responding Skills," 93—102.

2. Neimeyer and Bridges, "Postmodern Approaches to Psychotherapy," 298.

Part 2: Reflections and Theories

a calm, non-judgmental tone of voice. These practices or "common factors" also typically extend to all psychotherapy modalities, whether depth, humanistic, or postmodern.

A comment written many centuries ago in the Talmud (*Nedarim* 40a), explains that when we visit a sick person, we take away one sixtieth of that person's illness. The Talmud's comment doesn't get to the roots as to the *why* the visit to a sick person has healing power, but it does underscore the notion that pain and suffering potentially can shift in measurable ways, even a little bit—a sixtieth—when we are attentive to others who are ill. In more recent years, researchers are completing studies linking spiritual care with better health outcomes. Such "evidence-based" studies are getting increasing attention.[3]

As noted, individuals interested in developing more listening skills can consult the ample resources out there on techniques and tips. What isn't as easy to find are theories as to why listening is so powerful; that is, what happens in the listening encounter that promotes healing?

The next two sections seek to respond to this question. In Chapter XII, I respond from an anthropological point of view, with a focus on broad humanistic conditions. In Chapter XIII, I take a theological point of view where I share what I believe is at the core of listening's power as an experience that nurtures and comforts the spirit.

---

3. Lichter, "Studies Show Spiritual Care Linked to Better Health Outcomes."

XII.

Anthropology of Listening

WHILE ANTHROPOLOGY, THE STUDY of human societies and cultures, would encompass religion and theology, this section focuses on broader humanistic considerations. It addresses how the potency of listening engages us at sociobiological and neurological levels, and by means of widespread human values. A section offering a theology of listening, more specifically, follows.

THREE DEGREES OF INFLUENCE

Sociobiologically, listening to another connects us beyond the individual immediately in front of us. With the objective of establishing a warm, trusting, and safe connection, care providers impact the wider network of individuals influencing a patient's care. That is, our one-to-one relationships extend to influence the tenor of a patient's next tiers of relationships—evidently up to three degrees (at least).[1] In applying this three-degree-of-influence concept to listening, if a patient feels calmer, more at peace, less lonely as a result of being listened to deeply, this will impact those with whom the patient subsequently interacts. In other words, the next rings of caregivers or family members, in turn would be expected to

---

1. Christakis and Fowler, *Connected: The Surprising Power of Our Social Networks and How They Shape Our Lives,* 26–30.

become better equipped to care for the patient, being themselves calmer and more at peace.

Here's an example of how the theory of three degrees of influence might apply: My calming encounter with patient "Bert" spreads calm to his son Peter. Peter's greater calm spreads to his partner Dave, who is the one responsible for taking Bert to medical appointments. A few hours after my visit with Bert, he is not ready for Dave at the designated time for transport to his appointment. The theory is that Dave will be more patient toward Bert than he otherwise would have been, without that original visit between Bert and me. While the lasting effect of three-degree influences is not fully understood, it appears that at some level when we bring healthfulness of mind, emotion, body, and spirit to patients, the patients not only can "catch" this benefit from us, but they can spread it, too!

SOCIAL CONNECTEDNESS

Research demonstrates that social connectedness enhances our recovery from disease and increases our lifespan. Being married, having close family and friends, and belonging to and actively participating in social and religious groups significantly boosts our physical health.[2] One of the perks of the social connectedness involved in close relationships is the qualitative listening that takes place. Ideally this kind of listening reflects what transpires in caregiving relationships, and thereby can be an important component of the healing process.

In the vignette "Genevieve: Mirroring Empathy," in Part One, I make reference to the effect of "mirroring," and how one's own mirror neurons are said to "light up" parallel to certain actual experiences of others. My observation has been that when I listen attentively and non-anxiously to patients, more often than not, their own anxiety will lessen. In essence, they will begin to "mirror" me.

---

2. Goleman, *Social Intelligence*, 247.

EMOTIONAL CONTAGION

A similar concept is the phenomenon of *emotional contagion*, also previously mentioned—the concept purporting that humans can "catch" each other's emotions. Applied to caregiving, this would mean that patients can "catch" a caregiver's emotions; that is, our own centered, non-anxious presence, and thus reap positive, healthful effects for themselves.

HORMONES AND NEUROTRANSMITTERS

In recent years, many studies have reported on the optimal functioning in our bodies of hormones and neurotransmitters—oxytocin, cortisol, endorphins, dopamine, serotonin, and norepinephrine, to name a few. Oxytocin often is referred to as the "bonding hormone" because of the important role it plays in the neuroanatomy of intimacy. Following positive social interactions, oxytocin increases, contributing to measurable improvements in well-being. Cortisol, a steroid hormone released in response to fear or stress, can trigger the impulse to fight, flee, or freeze. Too much build-up of this substance can wreak havoc on our mental and physical health. Social connectivity is said to be one strategy that helps counter the effects of elevated cortisol.

High-quality caregiving would seem to support the optimal functioning of oxytocin, cortisol, as well as the other hormones and neurotrasmitters just named. For example, in reassuring caregiving encounters, presumably oxytocin increases—calming and helping to alleviate anxiety and feelings of chaos, and thereby assisting patients in coping, compliance, and cooperation. Presumably also, such supportive encounters can help lower cortisol levels; and lower cortisol levels means decreased experience of stress.

THE NERVOUS SYSTEM

Another biological dimension to consider is the nervous system. The *parasympathetic nervous system* (PNS)—having to do with

Part 2: Reflections and Theories

"rest, reflect, and digest"—is one of three main divisions of the autonomic nervous system (ANS). The two others are the *sympathetic nervous system* (actions requiring quick responses: fight, flight, freeze) and the *enteric nervous system* (gastrointestinal). In a calming and comforting care session, the PNS would be more engaged, allowing a patient to process difficult emotions more effectively and draw upon the "model" (calm) experience with the caregiver to anchor him or herself when later encountering more agitated circumstances. What we know about quality listening, *and* optimal functioning of biological substances and processes, suggests that a convergence of these realms would contribute greatly to health and healing.

According to a 2014 study in Canada, listening literally heals.[3] The researchers examined treatments for relief of chronic back pain—interventions carried out by physical therapists. Half the patients in the study who received a "sham treatment" (mild electrical stimulation) reported a 25 percent reduction in pain level. Patients who received the authentic electrical stimulation treatment did better, with pain levels decreasing by 46 percent. These two groups again were divided in half. The physical therapists provided one half of these patients with limited conversation. The therapists asked the other half open-ended questions, listened attentively to the answers, expressed empathy, and offered words of encouragement.

A summary of the study highlights the astounding findings: "Patients who underwent sham treatment but had therapists who actively communicated reported a 55 percent decrease in their pain.... Communication alone was more effective than treatment alone (46 percent relief). The patients who got [authentic] electrical stimulation from engaged physical therapists were the clear winners, with a 77 percent reduction in pain." This is an "evidence-based" example of how listening and good communication makes a measurable difference in the healing process!

---

3. Ofri, "The Conversation Placebo."

TRANSCENDENT INTEGRATION

Moving now to an example of how the potency of listening engages human values, I turn to a concept I call *transcendent integration*—a concept I would posit as reflecting a universal aspiration. Focusing more on a derived connotation rather than a traditional definition, I see transcendence as intimating: perspective, the long view, possibility, hope, transformation, and connectedness to meaning beyond the constrictions of one's current circumstances. I understand personal integration to include: self-awareness, self-knowing, self-acceptance, self-love, settledness within, insight, and being centered within oneself.

In listening attentively to our patients, we can support them as they cultivate transcendent integration. We can encourage them to fully engage their longing to reach out toward a reality or source of meaning that inspires expansion of consciousness beyond their own individual "bubbles." In the other direction, we can affirm their desire for inner peace.

To do these things is to journey with them in their struggle to touch into transcendent integration. This experience is one of harmony between the "out there" and the "in here"—between meaningful relationships, events, and objects that exist outside of themselves—*and* being present to and accepting of their internal, here-and-now experience. The gift of listening can help pave the way toward this harmony.

XIII.

A Theology of Listening

REFLECTING THE HUMAN LONGING to be listened to, sacred scriptures from many traditions present abundant examples of human beings crying out to God. In Hebrew Scriptures, over the course of Psalms' 150 chapters, the Psalmist calls out to God, expressing joy, anger, sorrow, vindictiveness, confusion, alienation, hope, gratitude, and more. Centuries later, Jesus on the cross famously quotes Psalm 22:1, crying out, "My God, my God, why have You forsaken me?" (Matt 27:46). A whole biblical book, "Lamentations," is identified with exactly that—lament, bitter and despair. Job, in the book about his trials, expresses despair and confusion about the tragedies that befall him. In Song of Songs, a whole different range of emotions emerges—including love, passion, desire, and longing.

From the tradition of Hinduism comes a parallel pattern. Hindu texts and myths contain vivid expressions of emotion by both humans and gods. Rama is the seventh avatar of the Hindu god Vishnu, and king of an ancient Indian city. Various scenarios in the *Mahabharata* describe Rama as filled with sorrow, grief, and agitation (263.23); pained by the arrow of love (264.4); and dispirited (266.4), among other emotions.[1] A fundamental Hindu spiritual work, the *Bhagavad Gita* (also a chapter in the *Mahabharata*), records an extended conversation between the human

1. Scharf, *Ramopakhyana—The Story of Rama in the Mahabharata*, 8.

Arjuna and Krishna/God. Arjuna pines, "My will is paralyzed, and I am utterly confused.... What can overcome a sorrow that saps all my vitality?" (2.7 and 2.8). Arjuna trusts that he can safely pour out his heart to God.

GOD IS WITH US

These examples provide illustrations of expressing emotion honestly and vulnerably before God. The inferred invitation is that God is prepared to receive us unconditionally, to accept us as we are, as this verse affirms: "When you call me, and come and pray to me, I will listen to you" (Jer 29:12). We can be sad or angry, joyful or grateful, vindictive or desirous. It doesn't mean we are off the hook in terms of growing in character. There are protocols for self-improvement in every major religion. Underneath the laws, precepts, and protocols for cultivating personal ethical qualities is the treasured experience of God as Emmanuel, or Imanu-El, literally "God with us." Much of the potency of Christian faith comes from the belief that God suffers with us, an idea with roots in Judaism. One who suffers with us implies a God who hears us and accepts us—in all of our darkness and in all of our light. Jewish and Christian traditions, among others, teach that at the baseline and for the long haul, God is with us, in whatever state we find ourselves. God fully knows and understands our suffering, as God suffers right alongside us.

HUMAN ENCOUNTERS CAN TAKE ON SPIRITUAL DIMENSIONS

As God allows full and free expression of a range of emotions, to the degree that chaplains and other caregivers emulate that invitation, the human encounter takes on a spiritual dimension. In truly listening, we invite others to an experience of feeling accepted in their full expression of themselves. That "blessing" can bring peace, reassurance, hope, self-compassion, and/or forgiveness (of self or others). Welcoming others to this sacred space of loving acceptance can inspire a feeling of being realigned with one's own truth and encourage a sense of freedom. This is the freedom that comes with being true, known, and seen before God; and the freedom that comes with embracing one's authenticity. The poet e.e. cummings captures this sentiment well:

> We do not believe in ourselves until someone reveals that something deep inside us is valuable, worth listening to, worthy of our trust, sacred to our touch. Once we believe in ourselves we can risk curiosity, wonder, spontaneous delight or any experience that reveals the human spirit.[2]

LIFTING UP OTHERS' SENSE OF WORTHINESS AND VALUE

Another transformation, with theological implications, that may happen in the process of listening is the lifting up of others' sense of worthiness and value. When chaplains and other caregivers see beyond an individual's current limits and troubles, and beyond the darker shadows lurking in his or her life story, they can affirm that within each human there is infinite worth and value. Those are qualities typically associated with what we might call the "Divine spark." In attuning ourselves to the essence of Divinity within the ones before us, we align with the theology of humans created in the Image of God. More poetically, we might say that our souls are God's breath. This theology implies that as much as the belief holds that God is surrounding us or is somewhere out there in the Universe, that God is within us, as well.

When we affirm, either explicitly or through our way of being present, that we perceive God's image in others—conveying that through how we listen, see, and attend to them—they may begin to see and embrace for themselves that sense of Divinity that resides within. Connecting to the Divine within means internalizing God's constant Presence. God shifts from "somewhere out there"

---

2. e.e. cummings, "Good Reads—Quotes."

to as close to us, as intimate, as our next breath. Potentially, such an experience can be a huge comfort, as well as a source of spiritual equanimity and a salve for existential loneliness, impacting healing on every level—physical, emotional, and interpersonal. In sum then, when we listen we have an opportunity to light a candle for another to see their Divine essence within. Attentive listening indeed can be spiritual care.

XIV.

Final Thoughts

DEAR CAREGIVERS: MY HOPE for this book is that it supports you through offering inspiration, affirmation, appreciation, and understanding for the work you do, for the comfort you provide, and for the healing you bring. Ideally through this support I offer you, the patients you serve will benefit as well. While I offer my own reflections, suggestions, tools, and possible interventions, your task is to embrace those ways of interacting that are most authentic to you and that evolve most organically in the caregiving relationship that is before you.

Caregiving challenges us to be nimble. We are called upon to be skilled *and* willing to engage spontaneous inspiration, humble *and* confident, knowledgeable *and* cautious about certainty, decisive *and* open-minded, clear *and* curious. The more we can remain attentive and responsive to the constantly evolving present moment, the more gratifying our work will be, and the more connected we will feel to those we care for.

When you care for another, you journey with that person. As you journey, may peace be upon you: Go in peace, be blessed with peace, and return in peace.

Bibliography

Brown, Brené. "Brené Brown on Blame," RSA video. https://www.youtube.com/watch v=RZWf2_2L2v8.

Christakis, Nicholas A., and James H. Fowler. *Connected: The Surprising Power of Our social Networks and How They Shape Our Lives—How Your Friends' Friends' Friends Affect Everything You Feel, Think, and Do.* New York: Back Bay Books, 2011.

Crumm, David. The Ram Dass Interview: Smiling as He Teaches About 'Polishing the Mirror.'" *Read the Spirit.* (July 14, 2013.) http://www.readthespirit.com/explore/the-ram-dass-interview-on-polishing-the-mirror-you-cant-help-but-smile-hes-still-teaching-us/.

cummings, e.e. Good Reads—Quotes. http://www.goodreads.com/quotes/7161-we-do-not-believe-in-ourselves-until-someone-reveals-that.

Freeman, Susan. "Jasmina: The Little Things." In *Reflective Practice: Formation and Supervision in Ministry,* Vol 37, May 2017.

Goleman, Daniel. *Social Intelligence: The New Science of Human Relationships.* NY: Bantam, 2006.

Gouldman, Graham and Eric Stewart, "The Things We Do for Love." Lyrics © Schubert Music Publishing, Inc, 1976. http://www.metrolyrics.com/the-things-we-do-for-love-lyrics-10cc.html.

Groves, Richard F., and Henriette Klauser. *The American Book of Living and Dying: Lessons in Healing Spiritual Pain.* Berkeley, CA: Celestial Arts, 2009.

Kabat-Zinn, Jon. "Meditation Quote 35: 'The little things? The little moments? They aren't little.'" http://dailymeditate.com/meditation-quote-35-the-little-things-the-little-moments-they-arent-little-jon-kabat-zinn/.

Kidd, Robert A. "Foundational Listening and Responding Skills." In *Professional Spiritual and Pastoral Care: A Practical Clergy and Chaplain's Handbook,* 92–103, Stephen B. Roberts, ed. Woodstock, VT: SkyLight, 2012.

Bibliography

Kornfeld, Jack. *Buddha's Little Instruction Book,* New York: Bantam, 1994.

Lichter, David A. "Studies Show Spiritual Care Linked to Better Health Outcomes." *Health Progress.* 94:2 (March-April 2013) 62–66. https://www.chausa.org/publications/health-progress/article/march-april-2013/studies-show-spiritual-care-linked-to-better-health-outcomes.

Neimeyer, Robert A., and Sara K. Bridges, "Postmodern Approaches to Psychotherapy." In *EssentialPsychotherapies, 2nd Edition*, edited by Alan S. Gurman and Stanley B. Messer, 149–77. New York: The Guilford, 2005.

Nitya, Brahmacharini. "Living Your Practice: Meditation in Action." In *Yoga International Special Edition: "Yoga for Busy Lives"* (2015) 101–3.

Norris, Kathleen. "Spirituality & Health." http://www.spiritualityhealth.com/quotes/peace—was-other-name-home.

Ofri, Danielle. "The Conversation Placebo," Sunday Review Opinion. *New York Times,* Jan. 19, 2017. https://www.nytimes.com/2017/01/19/opinion/sunday/the-conversation-placebo.html.

Pantanjali. "The Online Study Resource for the Yoga Sutras of Pantanjali." http://www.athayoganusasanam.com.

Remen, Rachel Naomi. "In the Service of Life." In *Noetic Sciences Review*, 37 (Spring 1996).

Scharf, Peter. *Ramopakhyana—The Story of Rama in the Mahabharata: A Sanskrit Independent-Study Reader.* London: Routledge, 2014.

Tillich, Paul. *Systematic Theology.* Chicago: The University of Chicago Press, 1967.

Yalom, Irvin D. *The Gift of Therapy: An Open Letter to a New Generation of Therapists and Their Patients.* NY: Harper Perennial, 2002.

www.ingramcontent.com/pod-product-compliance
Lightning Source LLC
Chambersburg PA
CBHW071438160426
43195CB00013B/1954